Blossoms from the Kalatuchi Tree

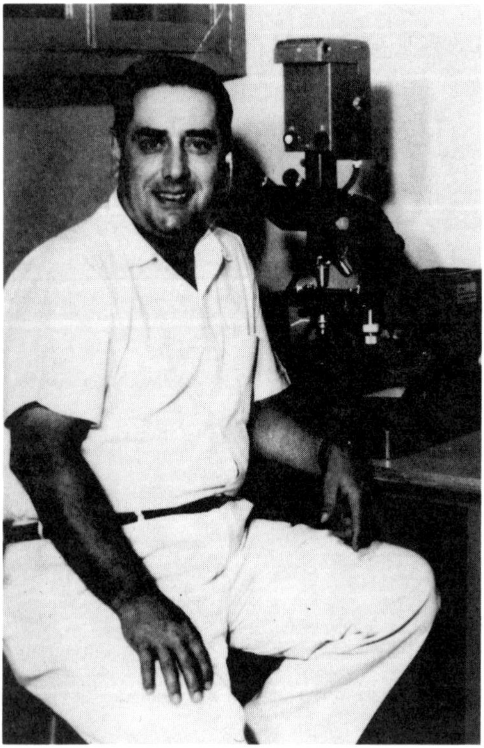

"It is my fondest hope that the memories that are so interesting to me in the early hours of morning are equally entertaining to others in the cold light of day." Claude V. Reich

Blossoms from the Kalatuchi Tree

Claude V. Reich

Claude V Reich

VANTAGE PRESS
New York • Los Angeles

FIRST EDITION

Published by Vantage Press, Inc.
516 West 34th Street, New York, New York 10001

Manufactured in the United States of America
ISBN: 0-533-09075-X

Library of Congress Catalog Card No.: 90-90109
0 9 8 7 6 5 4 3 2 1

This journal is dedicated to the three people who made it possible:

Val and Kim, my wife and daughter, who shared these experiences with me. The "Blossoms" were not all from a bed of roses, but their love made it seem that way.

Mrs. Antonio Madarang, Monina, whose life as my right arm, administrative officer, and private laboratory technician made my professional life easier and whose recent, far too early death made these memories much more painful.

And to:

The patients of Eversley Childs Sanitarium, Mandaue, Cebu, Philippines. For many years they have and still continue willingly to participate in investigations that they hope will lead to some relief for other people with leprosy throughout the world.

Contents

Foreword—to Sleep: Perchance to Dream

The easiest time of the day to understand the difference between dreaming and reminiscing occurs at three o'clock in the morning. That is also the most emotionally difficult time of the day. God, three o'clock in the morning is lonely! Nothing is moving. Life seems suspended in the blackness of space. When one awakens at three o'clock, one is forced to think, and all thoughts are magnified with a clarity not felt at any other time of the day. One can find a solution to any problem at three A.M. The normal becomes superior and the superior sublime.

Pains of the body and mind undergo the same mental amplification. At three A.M. all of the day's unpleasantness returns, and the pain that one struggled to bear in the daylight has been honed to a razor sharpness. The only escape one has is to take a flight into either fantasy or memory. To dream or to reminisce—either can be used to divert the mind from its otherwise unhindered intent to dwell on painful reality.

One must select that act of fancy or relive that part of the past that comes easily enough to the mind and is pleasant enough to induce the mind to put aside the pain of the day. The choice, fantasy or memory, is usually decided by age. The old have their memories which are both compensation and penalty for aging. Fantasy belongs mostly to the young. Fact and fancy are important at any age, but as one grows older, one accumulates more and more memories and the need for and significance of a mental lapse into fancy declines. Dreams lack the substance of a memory. The mind creates the emotion that accompanies a dream, but a memory carries within itself the record of the emotional reality of its own creation. Fantasy for the elderly is mostly a fanciful alteration of memory, to ease its pain, to make it more bearable.

I am a midnight muser. Too often I am forced to find an alternative to staring into the night and reliving the day just passed. Fortunately, I have more than enough wonderful memories of my life in Cebu, Philippines. These can be recalled with little effort and become a delightful escape from the reality of three o'clock in the morning. They also became the text that follows. It is my fondest hope that the memories that are so interesting to me in the early hours of morning are equally entertaining to others in the cold light of day.

Claude V. Reich, 1990

Blossoms from the Kalatuchi Tree

One

Lazarus, Come Forth

It seems that man has been in constant pursuit of knowledge of, or dominance over, anything that cuts his life shorter than he would like it to be. For most of human history, the lifespan of the human species was at the mercy of nature. In due course, man managed to conquer and control all visible enemies, except himself. However, those things that caused mankind the most grief, the great plagues and epidemics that decimated his ranks, were too complicated to have an easy answer.

There can be little doubt that quite early after the curse of free thought began to trouble the human mind, it began to seek an explanation for these sudden, wholesale episodes of death within human communities. With little to go on, it was only possible to resort to imagination. In the absence of any knowledge to the contrary, there could be little argument against the conception that these disasters were visited upon mankind by either jealous or vengeful gods or goddesses. The same logic that explained a plague must also cover a multitude of individual illnesses with equal acceptability, because once the primary axiom had been confirmed, the further truth becomes evident by default. Wherever an individual was ill there was little difficulty in finding some evidence that he alone had offended one or another of the many deities. Cause was easy to establish—if the community suffered, the community must have sinned; for an individual, the sin spoke for itself. Since the punishment was divinely intended, far be it for man to interfere. "Send him out from the camp" was man's penalty for leprosy, a sin made evident by lifelong sores and disfigurement—a certain sign from the gods.

While this science of the past seems rather primitive, it was a search for an explanation using a logical consideration of the knowledge that was available at the time. Today's medical science has benefited from the concept of a "germ theory of disease," but should be somewhat humble about the early development of this sacrilegious proposal that disease resulted not from gods, but from living things that were too small to see. The value of the "germ theory" was as controversial in its beginning as the concept of a divine cause for leprosy is today. Medical science has explained and brought the great plagues, epidemics and even most minor illnesses of mankind under control. As a result of this progress, it has been seen that the species of man has greatly multiplied and that all things born of woman have been invested with a longer and longer time to remain on this earth.

Within the communities of the human race, in spite of the major advances within the science of medicine, some people still die earlier than others. People are prone to question the necessity for early death, and societies are formed to promote research in the medical sciences to eliminate the causes for this premature death in the future. This phenomenon, for discussion purposes, could be called "premature death syndrome" (PDS). PDS must be eliminated, and, hence, PDS becomes the next challenge, the ultimate challenge, of medicine.

This tongue-in-cheek approach to the discussion of medical science is helpful if one wishes to explore the ultimate destiny of the discipline. Scientific research can only function on the supposition of an eventual successful solution to the problem in question. As each new agent of PDS is attacked by the scientific minds, one must assume that, as in the past, science will continue to succeed, and life will constantly be further prolonged. The ultimate goal can only be the day when the government proudly announces that all known causes of premature death have been discovered and eliminated. The health of the nation's people is now absolute. Everyone lives to his or her full biological life span. Medical science, funded by the National Institute of Health, is now working on the remaining problem, that a moderate variation, most likely genetic, in lifespan still exists between individuals. All persons should have an equal period on this earth, and genetic engineering is being applied to this final unfair circumstance that still exists in public health.

The government is most eager to solve the problem of unequal mortality since this variation also disturbs the national preset computer lifespan integrator which in turn complicates taxing policies and delays budget completion. In the Congressional hearings that will review the facts surrounding this problem, it will be discovered that PDS has not been totally resolved. For example, it has been disclosed that leprosy still exists in remote areas around the world. Medical science had failed to find a solution to this problem. To avoid any conflict between this age-old infection and the dramatic gains that were being made in the solution of PDS, the leprosy patient had been placed in communities of his own and isolated from the general view. Everyone will be amazed that this old disease, said to have existed in biblical times, is still prevalent in the world.

The events related above form an overstated scenario that is not too far beyond the realm of possibility. Most

Americans are amazed that, in the "high tech" era of science and medicine that exists today, the disease of leprosy remains as one of the major worldwide problems of human medicine. It has been estimated that as many as twenty million people throughout the world may be suffering from this infection. That figure sounds high, but if it is correct, it means that there are two people with this disease for about every three hundred people in the world. In the face of those numbers, how can it be possible that there are probably at least two hundred million Americans who have no idea that the disease still exists?

Leprosy is a subject of historical fear. By biblical description, it was a disfiguring disease that would not go away. It is unevenly distributed in the world. Since little could be done about it in the past, leprosy was easier to isolate than to acknowledge as a continuously unsolved problem. The unequal distribution of the disease not only makes it easier to isolate, but is also a facet of major importance in the continued failure to resolve this problem. Leprosy today is found mostly in those places where the money and the technology that are required to do the research are least available. Those people throughout the world who are concerned about this problem, and there are many, are confronted with the difficulty of trying to bring the people who suffer from leprosy together with the skills and instruments that are required to study the problem. That is not easy. To resolve the difficulty, is it easier to bring the mountain to Muhammad or Muhammad to the mountain?

The Leonard Wood Memorial, a foundation to raise funds to study leprosy, was named for the American who, as the governor general of the Philippines, gave not only his name, but much concern to this great problem in the territory that he administered. This foundation, one of the pioneers of modern medical research in leprosy, took

Muhammad to the mountain. One of the greatest of American men of science and probably one of the least known, Dr. H. Windsor Wade dedicated his life to an investigation of leprosy, and he did it on Culion, a small island at the western edge of the Philippines. At one time, this speck of land in the middle of nowhere, had more than seven thousand residents with leprosy.

There are more than seven hundred occupied islands in the Philippine archipelago. When one of the smallest and most remote of these has more cases of leprosy than all of the other islands combined there can be little question that a deliberate attempt is being made to remove these people from the human society. There also can be little question that, even in this remote part of the world, the attempt had been remarkably successful. Dr. Wade shared their isolation, studied their problem, reported on his studies, and in so doing brought them and leprosy to the attention of the world. He didn't solve the problems with a lifetime of devotion. He did help to enlighten the people of the rest of the world to the fact that leprosy, was not "out of sight, out of mind." Despite the fact that it had been so well hidden, it was still a problem and remained the responsibility of the world.

With Dr. Wade conducting research on Culion, the foundation then brought leprosy further out of its hiding place by establishing another leprosy care area on Cebu, a more central, more populated island closer to the society that breeds the problem. It was located only twelve miles north of the city of Cebu, an international seaport and the second largest city in the Philippines. The new sanitarium was named in honor of the American industralist, Eversley Childs, former president of the Bon Ami Corporation, who contributed all of the money that was required to acquire the land and to build the dormitories and administration buildings. Most people will remember Bon Ami, the scouring powder in the yellow can bearing the little yellow chick that "hasn't scratched yet."

Eversley Childs contributed even more additional money to staff and finance an international research program under the auspices of the Leonard Wood Memorial Foundation. Eversley Childs Sanitarium replaced the old "holding area" where, since Spanish times, newly discovered cases of leprosy had been accumulated to await transportation to Culion. Mr. Childs is long forgotten in his home country, but to this day his bust stands on a pedestal in the middle of the entrance road to Eversley Childs Sanitarium on the island of Cebu in the middle of the Philippines. It is there in recognition of his act of great charity.

The foundation later supported the construction of a laboratory and the development of a modern scientific research program within this new sanitarium. The building and furnishing of that laboratory, the hiring and training of staff and the development of research directed toward relief of leprosy were accomplished between 1962 and 1985, the twenty-three-year period of this narrative. Some of the events that occurred in that time became the memories that are the "Blossoms from the Kalatuchi Tree."

There was a long delay of thirty years between the establishment of the sanitarium and the building of the laboratory. The delay was the result of an economic depression with its subsequent effect on fund raising. Immediately following the depression came World War II, a world conflict that surrounded both Eversley and Culion. The war resulted in total neglect and unbelievable suffering on the part of leprosy patients in both of these institutions and probably everywhere in the world.

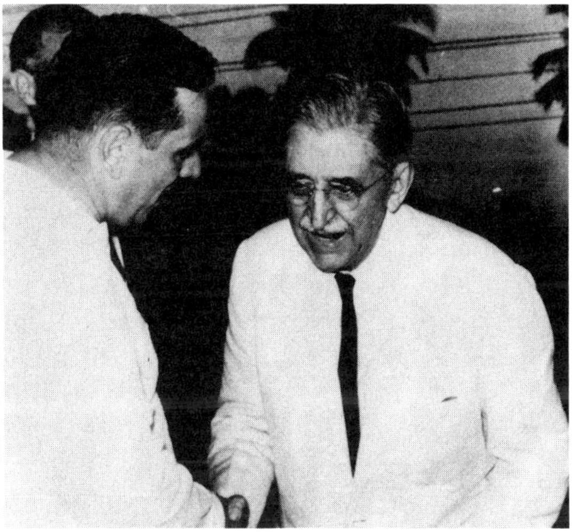

Dr. H. Windsor Wade dedicated his life to an investigation of leprosy, and he did it on Culion, a small island at the western edge of the Philippines.

Eversley was near the City of Cebu, so it experienced a contact relationship of sorts with the Japanese. Culion, an isolated island, was not bothered by the conquerors—it was completely ignored. The island is not nearly large enough and the soil is far too poor to support the large patient population that it had at the beginning of the war. When Culion and the rest of the Philippines came under Japanese domination, Dr. Wade remained behind with the patients; he shared their hunger and continued his research into the medical problem with the facilities and the materials that he had available. It was during this period that he could see and would later talk about the terrible effect of starvation on a person with this disease. It is somehow characteristic of leprosy research that it fails to attract its share of the scientific attention, but many of the workers that it does attract become totally dedicated, possibly because they become aware of the immensity of the problem and they share the social isolation of their subjects.

Leprosy is an infectious disease, but that statement should be made softly. It certainly does not appear to be a very infectious disease. Leprosy workers definitely do not deserve sainthood for the apparent risk that they assume when they associate with the leprosy patient. History shows that few, if any, leprosy workers ever contract the clinical disease. However, in spite of its low level of infectivity, it does spread slowly in the person in whom it appears. Therefore it is logical to assume that the disease must pass from one who has it to one who will get it. That process, by definition, makes it an infectious disease, but the procedure by which this transmission occurs remains uncertain.

The cause of the disease remains equally uncertain. Under the microscope one can see a potential invader in the tissues and fluids from sores of the disease. This object is a bacteria, not a virus which is far smaller and would not be visible under the light microscope. It is present in such enormous numbers that, without further scientific evidence, it is most logical to assume that it is the cause and not an effect. It is difficult to dispute the assumption that this entity causes the disease, but as a matter of scientific integrity, the bacteria in question must remain as a good bet, but not an absolute certainty, to be the cause. That statement sounds like a moot point, but the difference between a good bet and absolute certainty is as great as the difference between believing and knowing, between superstition and science—especially when the medical problem persists and the "good bet" assumption provides little help toward finding a solution to the problem.

Contrary to popular belief, leprosy does not cause the fingers, hands and feet to fall off. If uncared for, it does result in disability and deformity, but today these are more to be considered as results of neglect than as inevitable properties of the infection. Leprosy can be treated. There are several drugs that can be used to treat this disease. Two of these have been used alone over long periods of time and have been confirmed to be effective in arresting the disease, but most workers have hesitated to use the word "cure" for these drugs because there is evidence of long-term failure in many patients using them.

The other potentially effective drugs have never produced independent arrests, but they do have a theoretical effect based on laboratory data and have shown evidence of short-term clinical effects. One of these potential drugs has been combined with the two confirmed drugs into a multidrug therapy program which is said to bring about a cure for

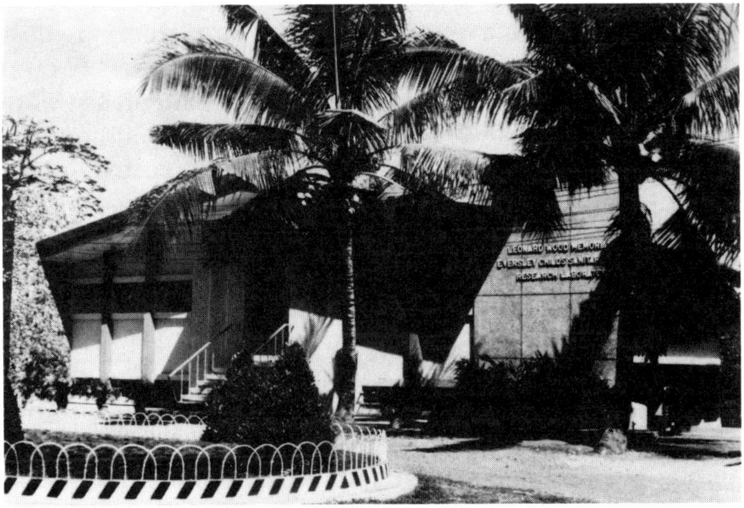

The laboratory—the building and furnishing of that laboratory, the hiring and training of staff and the development of research were accomplished within the twenty-three-year period of this narrative.

leprosy. The word "cure" is now being used, and so the multidrug treatment is said to be doing what none of the components can do alone. The multidrug effect appears to be an example of a total that is greater than the sum of its parts, which is a possibility in the treatment of disease. The large number of adherents to the multidrug program would lead one to believe that there is some substance to the use of the word "cure," but the past history of use of this word with leprosy would advise some caution for a few more years.

Cure or not, the real dilemma lies in the problem of applying the cure to the disease. Drugs are expensive and leprosy is mostly distributed in areas around the world where there are so many other problems that one wonders what priority can be given to leprosy. Leprosy treatment requires time. Even under the best of conditions, the multidrug program will require at least two years of dedicated therapy to effect the cure, and ideally there should be a constant followup for perhaps a minimum of ten years after that. That kind of dedication is difficult to achieve. However, even more difficult is the task of reaching the patient. Its widespread, uneven and low-level distribution throughout the world and the general, irrational fear of leprosy would make for extremely difficult accessibility to the disease.

Leprosy assumes many forms along a scale from benign to chronic progressive terminal. Even physicians skilled in the handling of the disease have had serious and loud disagreement over the diagnostic characteristics of the various forms. Unskilled physicians will most likely never diagnose leprosy except as the last possible diagnosis for a medical problem with which they are unfamiliar and which is not responding to their attention. A most interesting characteristic and one that is little known to the layman is the fact that leprosy as a disease does not progress from the benign to the terminal state. The benign form of leprosy, which in many areas of the world is the most frequent form, will heal itself. Even without any medical attention it is an unpleasant illness that will cause deformities, but will heal.

In biblical times leprosy was not wholly diagnosed by its appearance, but to a great extent by its persistence in the patient. If a person had sores that refused to disappear over a sequence of seven-day examinations by the priest, the sufferer was said to have leprosy. If, at any time after this pronouncement, his sores did heal to the priest's satisfaction, he was declared free from leprosy. Leprosy was the disease whose sores did not go away. During the period when the priest determined that the plague of leprosy was in the person, he was to "remain outside of the camp."

In medieval times this pronouncement was made with much greater severity. The person with leprosy was made to attend his own funeral service. A handful of earth was

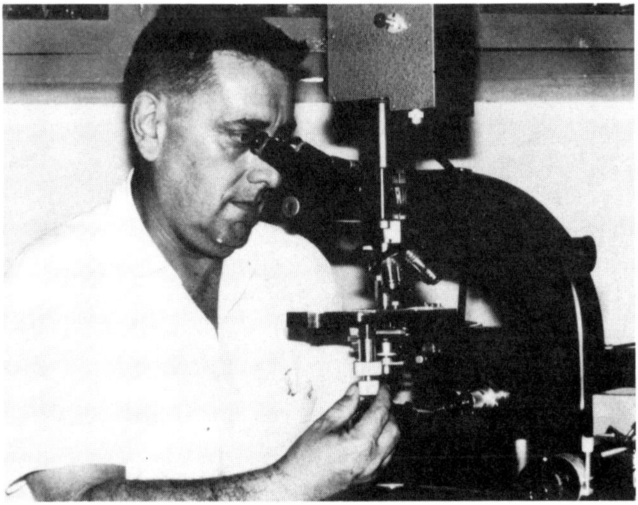

The microscope—the cause of the disease remains equally uncertain. Under the microscope one can see a potential invader in the tissue and fluids from sores of the disease.

tossed on his abode, as on a grave, and he was considered to be no longer of this earth. Even though he walked among them, at a safe distance, he and others like him were to have no further association with anyone except their own kind. Lazarus, of whom it was sometimes said that he had leprosy, became and still is the figure image of the leprosy sufferer, and St. George is the patron saint who slays the dragon representing leprosy.

In modern times the leprosy patient still suffers, not only from a bacterial infection, but also from painful social leftovers of the historical perception. Patients are still separated from society in many places in the world. As a result of this separation, the rest of the people in the world are not only ignorant of the relatively noninfectious nature of the disease, but they are not even aware that the problem still exists. Like any problem of any kind, it must be recognized as a problem in order to accomplish a solution. The people of the world must accept some responsibility for its existence.

It is not easy to find financial support for the studies that are required to know this disease well enough to resolve it. Leprosy is not likely to be the kind of condition that will complicate the lives of the families and friends of the powerful who must provide that support. The leprosy solution will be the result of the most charitable of all charities—help for strangers with a problem that can never be mine. You feel that by seeing the way they live, you believe that by listening to them, you become certain of that by loving them.

Two

A Quest to Prove a Cause: At Work

. . . persons suspected of the disease were first summoned before a priestly tribunal, and then sent for examination by two or more surgeons. If the surgeon declared it leprosy, the decree of separation was pronounced and read in the parish church. On the following Sunday the leper was fetched from his dwelling by a deputation of priests, laid on a funeral bier, and covered over with a black cloth; and in this manner was borne to the church, the priests chanting the "Libera Me." In the church the bier was placed upon trestles, and the leper lay there and listened to his funeral service, after which the congregation passed before him, sprinkling him with holy water, and each bestowing alms upon him. The service of the dead being completed, another funeral procession was formed, and with the cross going in front, the leper was carried to the hovel where he must live unvisited and unattended until death claimed him. Gloves, clappers, and a bread bowl were given to him by the priest, who cast over the hut a handful of earth from the cemetery, and the "De Profundis" was then sung.

"Dead to the world, be thou alive again to God," said the priest, and then bidding him to remember that the Church would be ever mindful of him in its prayers, the priest went on to pronounce sentence of deprivation: "I forbid thee to enter any church or monastery, any mill, bakehouse, or market, or any place in which there is a concourse of people; I forbid thee to walk with naked feet or to go out of thy dwelling without thy leper's garment and thy clappers; I forbid thee to wash thyself or anything thou hast in any river, stream or fountain; what water thou needest fill it into thy barrel with a bowl. I forbid thee to touch anything thou art bargaining for until thou hast bought it; I forbid thee to enter any tavern; I forbid thee if thou art spoken to in the street to make any answer until thou hast observed the direction of the wind; and I forbid thee to walk in narrow streets. I forbid thee to touch the well or the cord of the well with ungloved hands; I forbid thee to eat in any company save that of lepers like thyself; and I bid thee know that when thou diest thy body will be buried in this cavern and not in holy ground." This tremendous and blasting sentence being uttered, the priest planted a wooden cross before the door, hung on it a box for alms—and the leper was left alone.

This description of the "Ceremony of Separation," a religious ritual that was accomplished for centuries in medieval Europe was taken from a 1936 edition of the *International Journal of Leprosy*. The finality of this ceremony as a social response to a human problem has no counterpart in medicine and is indicative of the unique character that man assigned to this malady. Mankind lived with all of its other medical problems; leprosy alone was buried—alive.

Leprosy continues to be an enigma to this day, although thankfully without the medieval finality of symbolic death. Only a bit more than fifty years ago, a short time in the history of this disease, a man of science showed that a drug, a sulfone, had the capability to delay the course of this infection. Dr. Paul Faget, in the United States Public Health Service Hospital at Carville, Louisiana, reported that the disease did not progress in ten clinically advanced patients during one year of experimental therapy with this drug. In this report Dr. Faget led the world to a drug that became the first bona fide means in history to provide some medically logical comfort for the human misery caused by this disease. It is of special interest to note that the drug did not cure any of the experimental patients; it only stayed the advancement of the disease during the year of observation. This was hardly a solution, but certainly a ray of hope.

Today we know that the patient should expect a wait of about two years to see any noticeable improvement. It takes about five years until the disease appears to be under complete control. In spite of its delayed action, the drug commonly known as DDS (Diamino diphenyl sulfone) has been the main weapon in our handling of leprosy for almost fifty years. For most of that time it was the only weapon. There is one other drug available today that, given alone, can bring about the same kind of relief from leprosy. This drug, called Lamprene in Europe and Clofazimine in America, is discussed later in these memoirs as the "black medicine" in the story of a leprosy patient. That patient, Jose Ramos, also became a very good friend.

There are other drugs that are used in the handling of leprosy cases, but these drugs are rarely given alone. They are supplementary drugs, and their use is rationalized on the basis of laboratory conclusions. Their continued use is justified on the basis of an apparent short-term clinical benefit rather than on any demonstrated long-term, independent, curative effect. The major drugs, DDS and Clofazimine, are the only independently effective treatments available. These two drugs are the basis for our present-day cavalier attitude towards leprosy. They are not without their difficulties, but they are the tools that have brought leprosy out of the dark ages.

DDS and Clofazimine are prime examples of the enigma that surrounds leprosy. Both drugs were discovered as the result of experimental assumptions that most likely are not true. Drug trials in leprosy are time-consuming and very expensive. Many possible drugs are available, but there is no experimental means to screen these drugs to test their potential for the costly trials. Accordingly, test drugs were usually selected on the assumption that tuberculosis and leprosy are caused by related organisms. It was further assumed that any drug that is effective for tuberculosis should work for leprosy.

The sulfone was said to be effective for tuberculosis. It was tried for leprosy. It worked! The drug Clofazimine was one of a series of drugs that were designed for tuberculosis therapy. It was tried for leprosy. It worked! From these examples, it could be said that the experimental assumption is sound. However, after the effectiveness of DDS and Clofazimine was confirmed for leprosy, it was discovered that these two drugs were ineffective for tuberculosis. The phenomenon of reaching your goal by taking the wrong path is called "serendipity." Serendipity is another way of saying, "we were lucky" or even, "the Lord smiled on us." However that fact should not detract from the significance of the discoveries nor from the value of the findings.

The scientific problem is far more difficult than appears on the surface. Science is a matter of measures. There are only three experimental approaches to the problem. Measure the effect of the drug on the infected human. Measure the effect of the drug on an infected experimental animal. Measure what happens in the test tube when the drug is tested directly against the living entity that is causing the disease.

Again we are faced with the enigma of leprosy. The living entity that causes leprosy cannot be grown in the test tube. The scientist is faced with the choice of either using the animal or of tolerating the human misery. The answer must be obvious. Until another means is available, it is necessary to test the drugs in the animal. The cost as well as the ethics of this circumstance then dictates that it is essential to try all possible means to cultivate the germ that causes leprosy. When the leprosy organism is cultured, neither the animal nor man will need to be the primary experimental device.

The cause of leprosy is uncertain, and that is another part of the enigma. There is a bacterium that can be seen when one uses the microscope to observe tissues taken from a leprosy sore. This germ is not obvious in all leprosy tissues, but where it is found it seems to increase in numbers as the disease worsens. All observations indicate that this germ is associated with the disease, but it is not clear whether this germ alone can cause leprosy. No one has ever been able to transmit leprosy under the defined experimental conditions that are necessary to answer that question.

How does one prove what causes any disease? This question is basic to the science of microbiology. It was essential to the early revelation that germs, not gods, cause human disease. A German scientist named Robert Koch defined the scientific steps to prove cause. Koch's postulates stipulated that one first must isolate a suspected germ from the human patient and grow it outside of the body. One then must use the pure test tube growth to produce the identical disease in an experimental animal. From the sick animal, one must isolate and grow a germ that is identical to the original germ taken from the human patient.

It is easy to visualize the act of confirmation in this series of steps. This procedure, when properly followed, eliminates doubt and argument about a disease. Fear disappears with uncertainty. It has long been the accepted scientific procedure for determining the cause of disease. Koch followed these postulates to confirm the cause of tuberculosis, and as a result, there is little doubt or argument about that disease. Today, tuberculosis is still serious, but it is no longer the feared problem that it was in earlier times in human history.

There are certain similarities in the tuberculosis germ and in the microscopic bodies that can be seen in leprosy sores. For this reason, most leprosy workers consider the two life forms to be related. However, unlike tuberculosis, the germs that are seen in leprosy sores have never been confirmed as the cause of leprosy. It has not been possible to apply the series of steps that result in scientific proof because the germ that is said to cause leprosy has never been grown outside of the animal host.

I went to Cebu to isolate, confirm and study the cause of leprosy. It was my quest to shed light on a problem that has haunted mankind in almost every age of its history. I had the temerity to assume that I was worthy of the task. When I went to Cebu in 1962, the number of leprosy cases in the Philippines was estimated to be about twenty-nine thousand. On my last visit to Cebu in July 1983, that number was estimated to be fifty-five thousand. Those figures are proof that I did not succeed in my quest. I failed in my quest for the "grail," but I was fortunate enough to look upon it.

To culture the leprosy bacillus, what a marvelous goal. I wish that I had been given the time to really devote my full attention to this cause, but the foundation never gave me that opportunity. I had to build the laboratory, train the staff, supervise laboratory services for other leprosy projects throughout the world and keep account of the money. In whatever time I could find after these chores I was allowed to use the lab for my own scientific efforts. However, the foundation did not provide me with the funds to finance cultivation. I was expected to raise outside money to fund the microbiology research.

My goodness but this sounds sad. Occasionally, the injustice of my life would weigh me down, and I would pour out my heart to my staff. I had one technician who was one of the most marvelous listeners. Soori Bell, pronounced Surrey, could be profoundly attentive. At exactly the right moment, she would offer me sympathy by saying, loudly, "Poor baby!" The long lyric slur that she used to make this comment put my problems into proper perspective. One of the compensations that one receives from working with the leprosy problem is that there are many people around you with greater problems than yours. Try saying to a person with leprosy, "So you think you have problems, let me tell you about mine." It is very difficult to walk a mile in the shoes of the leprosy patient.

In spite of my protests, I did manage to accomplish a good amount of cultivation research during my career. I tried an unbelievable number of nutrients under an unbelievable number of conditions in an unbelievable number of test tubes. In addition, I attempted to repeat every report of cultivation by other workers whenever I had the means to do it accurately. No new patient that entered the Eversley Childs Sanitarium during my stay was allowed to receive one iota of medication before he was asked if he would be willing to submit a specimen for Dr. Reich's attempts to culture the leprosy bacillus.

When I ran out of incubator space for my thousands of test tubes, I had more incubator cabinets built. I never felt comfortable terminating any culture experiment. Leprosy is such a slow disease that the researcher can never be sure that growth will never appear in any given tube. When you are looking for a sign of life, any possible sign of life, from an organism under conditions in which no one has ever seen a sign of life it is impossible to say when to stop looking. For whatever kind of mentality it may ascribe to me, I doubt if there are many people in this world who spent as much of their lifetime looking through a microscope at bacteriologic smears of leprosy specimens as I did.

Since no one has ever grown the germ before, it is not known just what sign of life one must look for. The most obvious and the final arbiter of growth is multiplication, but it is not easy to tell if a germ is multiplying when the multiplication is so very, very slow. Counting germs is the basis of the science of microbiology. Leprosy is the ultimate challenge to that science.

There were many times when I was convinced that the tubes that I was observing at the moment had more leprosy germs in them than I had put in them at the beginning. I would go home elated with my success, ready to announce my profound discovery to the world. On those nights, I would bubble over to Val, my wife, about how simple the task of growing the leprosy germ really was when you finally achieved it and how stupid I had been for not seeing the solution earler. I rarely slept on those nights. I would be wide awake planning the marvelous experiments of discovery that will inevitably follow the culture of the leprosy agent.

I always returned to the lab the next day eager to repeat my triumphs, only to get results that were not quite as astounding as I expected. Usually on this second day my results were maddening, neither confirming nor denying yesterday's conclusions. On that, the post-success evening at home, I was usually tired from the long period of nervous anticipation and humbled by the doubt resulting from the questionable evidence of this day's experiments. I would sleep, but not well. In the next few days the results, always eventually the same, would reveal that the germs were not growing. In this way, life went from the highest of "highs" to the lowest of "lows," often overnight.

Val soon learned to take my first day's exuberance in stride, and she would caution me to wait for tomorrow's results. These recommendations, when followed, kept my spirits on a more even keel. However, I do remember at least one set of experiments that were so good that my high lasted for several weeks. The long low that followed taught me that in life as in science, for every force there is an equal and opposite force. What the hell, sometimes it is worth a long low to experience the profound feeling that accompanies a great success, even a short-term imaginary one.

In 1873, Armauer Hansen in Norway reported that he attributed the cause of leprosy to a bacteria, which he had observed and described. That report, in the early days of the germ theory, was the first ever to propose a germ as the cause of a specific human disease. In nearly every year of the more than one hundred years since Hansen's report, there has been at least one new report that someone, somewhere in the world of leprosy research has found the grail—has cultivated the cause of leprosy. This false promise has occurred so often in the scientific literature of leprosy research that today any report of successful cultivation is usually greeted with a yawn and the comment, "Well here is another one." The scientist who reports a successful cultivation of leprosy is like the little boy who cried wolf too often.

One year it happened in my laboratory at Eversley. I heard "through the grapevine" that no less than my Filipino technician was claiming that he had cultured the leprosy bacillus. I immediately called a staff meeting to question the truth of the rumor. My information was more than rumor; it was indeed true. Epiphanio confirmed that he had succeeded where all others had failed. When I requested that I should be given the details of this marvelous feat, I was told that the procedure could not be revealed until the report had been submitted for publication. It was feared that someone else may take the credit for the discovery.

Needless to say that as laboratory director, I did not take kindly to this situation. I ordered that no publications were to be made from the Leonard Wood laboratory without a proper evaluation of the contents by a committee of the author's peers. When I persisted in my demand for further information, I was informed that all of my Philippine colleagues, including the five doctors, had already reviewed and approved the paper.

I was also told that it was known that I had already taken credit for the discovery. As proof of this fact, I was shown an article in a news clipping from a recent scientific newsletter. The article stated that an American scientist had reported the successful tissue culture cultivation of the leprosy bacillus at a meeting in Washington, D.C. Since it was known that I had attended that meeting, it was assumed that I had made that report in Washington. They weren't sure how I did it, but they were certain that I had somehow discovered how Epiphanio had accomplished the task before I left for the meeting.

No one really believed my protests to the contrary. In fact, they were not interested in my explanation that "tissue culture cultivation," as described in the newsletter, and "culture from tissue" that they were supposedly doing were two completely different procedures. I tried to explain that the newsletter report was not about me and was in no way related to their so-called discovery. In spite of their unwillingness to accept my explanation, I stressed that I didn't care what they believed, no report would come out of this lab without a full evaluation of the data to see if it supported the conclusion.

Two days after this meeting the *Manila Times* carried an article stating that "American Scientist [is] Suppressing

Philippine Discovery." That article was followed up on successive days by reports on the marvelous Filipino discovery of the germ that causes leprosy. In the following week the Philippine secretary of health announced an investigation of the American who was suppressing Philippine science. That meant *me*!

A panel was quickly appointed to investigate me and that panel came to Cebu for the purpose. They selected my personal secretary, Fernando Arriola, to serve as recording secretary to the panel. Fed also happened to be the brother of one of the panel members. I was appalled, not by the obvious bias and jeopardy that this act imposed on me, but by the fact that I knew damned well that my secretary was not capable of taking notes from dictation. He had been hired for me before my arrival in Cebu. The political weight of his appointment to the job had made it impossible for me to object. I had to continue using him as my secretary in spite of a good number of shortcomings, not the least of which was a complete ignorance of shorthand. During the several years that he had worked for me, I had to do all of my writing in long hand. Fed then typed my notes and letters from my yellow legal notepads, slowly but beautifully.

I tried to make the panel aware of the doubt that I had about my secretary's ability to handle the chore of notetaking. Apparently all that I accomplished was to infuriate the panel member who was his brother. He in turn imparted his impatience with me to his fellow inquisitors. My objection to having Fed Arriola, my personal secretary, serve as secretary to the government panel that was investigating me was not exactly a smart move on my part. I finally resigned myself to the inevitable and agreed to let him record the events of the proceedings. To compound the injustice, the foundation paid his salary for this duty.

First thing next morning, I faced the "Committee to

Investigate American Suppression of Philippine Science." I took the position that I did not intend to suppress the publication. I only wished to have the report evaluated before it was published in order to save both the Leonard Wood Memorial and Philippine science from any possible embarrassment. I also informed the government that I was glad that I had taken this stance. We had now been able to prove that the germ that had been isolated by Epiphanio did not come from the leprosy patient, as it was reported. The germ that had been isolated came instead from the distilled water that was used in the preparation of the culture medium. I stressed that I had not been able to check this earlier because of the refusal on the part of my colleagues to inform me of their procedure. My position not to allow the use of the foundation's name on the publication had saved the foundation from embarrassment. I regretted that I had not been able to act quickly enough to stop the publication and save Philippine science also from the embarrassment of an inaccurate scientific report.

During this entire four-hour morning session, my secretary was making shorthand notes on a pad in front of him at a furious and apparently effortless pace. I was absolutely amazed and impressed. When the chairman called a halt to the morning's meeting, he thanked the secretary. With a side look toward me, he asked him to type as much of the proceedings as he could during the two-hour lunch break so that we could review the details in the afternoon session. There was little that I could do except apologize to Fed. I went to lunch, shaking my head all the way home and thinking, Damnit that guy has professed incompetency all this time simply to avoid work.

I took a long lunch and a leisurely siesta not knowing what was going to happen in the afternoon and not really caring. I did feel that I had acquitted myself well and that we would lay the problem to rest in the afternoon. When I later returned to the lab and my office, I found Fed in my office, sitting at my desk *behind closed doors* crying profusely. He didn't wait for me to ask for the reason. When he saw me, he immediately sobbed, "Dr. Reich, I don't know how to take shorthand."

The revelation made me catch my breath and finally I said, Why in the h——didn't you say that this morning? What were you doing with all that note scratching all morning?"

"I am sorry, *Dooktor*—I was afraid."

"Well now what do you intend to do?"

Now the tears became torrents and Fed sobbed even more wildly, "Help me, *Dooktor*."

I am sure that I must have vented some unrepeatable phrases in the moments that followed, but suddenly I became impressed with the comic opera character of the events that were unfolding around me. The entire scenario was unreal. I began to laugh and Fed, most likely thinking that I was going mad, began to sob even more. I said, "You wait here, somebody has to get this situation back to reality."

I left the room to look first for my secretary's older brother and next for the undersecretary of health to the Philippines who had been the panel chairman for the morning. Both of these individuals, when found and informed, went into my office where Fed was still sobbing. I remained outside waiting their decision. The decision, when it arrived, was a bit unusual, but in view of the situation not at all unbelievable. In fact it was probably the most logical turn of events for the day. The chairman informed me that, unfortunately, there were no notes available for the morning session, so it would be necessary to repeat the morning's investigation again this afternoon. Did I know where we could find another secretary, quickly?

The secretary of one of the Philippine doctors, also a foundation employee, was sent for and served to record the afternoon repeat session. This guy was good. Not only could he take notes, he typed so damned fast that he typed the entire session verbatim—without error. The situation was normal, it went from the ridiculous to the sublime without a pause. Nothing more was said about Fed's fallacy, the great shorthand fraud, but I knew that the older brother was going to have a lot to say to my secretary that evening.

The afternoon session of the investigating committee was almost a replica of the morning. I was aware that I could not afford a single contradiction of anything that I had said earlier. It was difficult to remember every facet of my morning testimony, but I tried and apparently succeeded. At the end of the afternoon session, we not only had an immediate typewritten record, but the chairman exonerated me and apologized in the name of the Philippine people. That apology and a short description of the panel findings later appeared as a small article on the back pages of the *Manila Times*.

Apology be damned, there is a scientific report in "The Journal of the Philippine Leprosy Association" reporting the isolation and successful cultivation of the cause of leprosy. The report is completely without fabric. It is one of the great failures of human science that published scientific mistakes remain in the journals forever. The corrections, if they are made, are always in some other location, and reference to them is usually lost or difficult to find.

The report of my colleagues has never been corrected in the literature. It will have no further role in the answer to the leprosy problem. Its continued presence in the literature will stand as an indicator of the great value that the leprosy worker assigns to the isolation of the cause of leprosy. To culture the leprosy bacillus is like finding gold. You want to get it into the bank before you let anyone know you have it for fear they will steal it from you. This particular report is not alone; it is one of too many such reports that clutter the leprosy literature. These reports make the effort even more complicated than it should be. Neither my name nor the name of the foundation is on the report, but I still get angry about the fact that it was all so unnecessary. I resent the great amount of my time that it took away from the work that I really wanted to do. I never cultivated the cause of leprosy. I didn't capture the grail, but I sure learned to bear a few crosses during my search.

Three

A Lay Lesson in Leprosy: Dalmacia

I doubt that I'll ever forget the first time that I entered the leprosarium. I was an experienced microbiologist on the staff of The Johns Hopkins University, so the act should have been of little significance to me. It surprised me when, in spite of myself, I felt the hairs on the back of my neck rising. There was a warmth to my breath that had nothing to do with the tropical climate. I found myself trying to avoid any appearance of staring at people, and yet I was curious. I had seen leprosy before, but this time I was going into a place where it resided. Good intentions be damned, I stared at everyone during the entire walk of about five hundred yards between the entrance at the main road and the site of the new laboratory. Deep inside of me was an anticipation that was unnerving and strange. I wanted to see the horrible markings that this terrible disease inflicted on the unfortunate residents of this darkened place of isolation.

Instead, I saw nothing unusual. The stroll up the hard packed earthen road became a lovely walk along a flowering hibiscus hedge, under a canopy of palm trees bearing clusters of coconuts. Very ordinary people were tilling corn in a sunlit field along the lower side of the road, and laughing children ran past me. I saw not a mark on a single child. Some of the children even had the audacity to be singing when everything inside of me said that they should be moaning. I saw no horrible faces, only smiling ones. Everyone that I passed—everyone—said, "Good morning, Doctor" as if they meant it. I was thrilled to know that they were aware of my coming and knew who I was. Before I reached the laboratory, I was completely taken up by a beauty that I never expected. The leprosarium was beautiful then. I don't ever recall it being not beautiful.

Ahead of me at the top of the slow incline of the entrance road, I could see the slight plateau that was the center and the highest spot of the institution. Here, the road branched. The right branch led to the director's residence and continued past that to the home of the Belgian nuns who were volunteer help in the institution and guests of the Philippine government. At this point the right branch ended abruptly. In fact it ended so abruptly that any car progressing to this house of the Sisters of the Immaculate

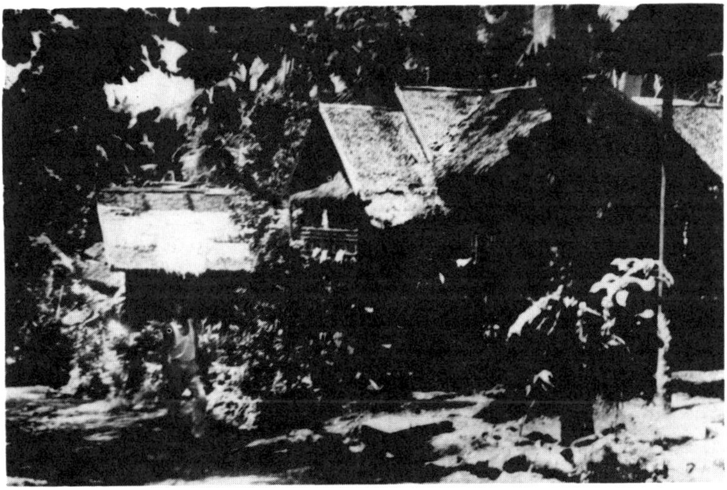

From there I could look slightly down onto the nipa-thatched homes of the tropical campus stretched out before me in the sunlight.

Conception of Mary had to back out for lack of space in which to turn around.

On the left branch around a long curve, just past the ghost tree, were the administration buildings and across from them was the site of the new laboratory. From the rear of the laboratory one could see the rear of the house of the nuns and a footpath that these elderly ladies of mercy used to walk past the laboratory and down into the hospital grounds itself. From the front of the laboratory, I could look slightly down onto the nipa-thatched homes and white-painted metal roofs of the tropical campus stretched out before me in the sunlight. The clear blue sky that was over me was filled with wispy white clouds. It looked strangely like the same sky that was over the people on the outside.

There are many, with much knowledge of leprosy, who insist that the biblical manifestation called leprosy and the disease that bears this name today are not the same. They insist that the unwarranted fear of leprosy is the result of centuries of conditioning to a biblical association that is unjustified. They base their argument on the observation that the description of leprosy from Leviticus in the Bible does not match the medical description of the leprosy seen today.

There is no question in my mind that the general attitude that leprosy is the ultimate in horrible diseases is completely unjustified. There is no question that the fear of leprosy is unwarranted; however, I have never been able to convince myself that this disease is not the leprosy of the Bible. To me, the biblical description does and yet does not fit. I'll leave that argument to the experts. The problem I have with the argument is contained in the simple question, if the people of the Bible did not call this disease leprosy, what did they call it? It is almost certain that the disease that I am seeing today did exist then.

Regardless of its name, it is certain that the general fear of leprosy is irrational. The general concept of leprosy is unreal. People who have never seen the disease and who have no idea whatsoever of its nature can be most intolerant to the unfortunate sufferer of this affliction. I don't ascribe their intolerance of an unfortunate person who needs their understanding to a fear resulting from the description of leprosy that they have read in the Bible. I credit their intolerance to their failure to practice the understanding that they may have read about in the Bible.

Leprosy is not quarantined in the Philippines. The leprosarium called Eversley Childs Sanitarium, after its American donor, is not a confinement institution. There are no walls or locked gates. The only fence is a low wire obstacle that functions mostly as a boundary marker. Neither is Eversley Childs Sanitarium really a sanitarium. The word does not fit. It is a word that implies an isolation that is inconsistent with current practice, or practicality, in leprosy care. "Sanitarium" is a word that disturbs my sensibility. It is an earlier word that was used to avoid use of the term "leprosarium." I will continue to use the word leprosarium for this narrative, but the time is now ripe to discard both terms. Eversley Childs is a hospital.

Most leprosy patients in the Philippines are treated at outpatient clinics and remain living at home. Institutions like Eversley Childs care for those who for social or economic reasons, or because of age or neglect at home, need special attention. Eversley is an institution that offers evidence of man's humanity to man. Its cluster of buildings, dormitories and individual residences nestles among the surrounding outside homes and villages like an exclusive residential subdivision. The hospital residents and those of the surrounding communities intermingle in many areas of endeavor. The organized hospital entertainment is quite popular with the outside neighbors. They are welcome to attend and do. There is no evidence whatsoever that this cohabitation has ever caused grief to the neighborhood. No one gets leprosy from the hospital; they get leprosy in some as yet uncertain manner outside of the hospital and then are admitted as members of the patient community.

Only a few of the residents, perhaps less than ten percent, need special bed care attention in either the small male or the smaller female infirmary. This group of bed patients usually includes a good number who are temporarily confined for reasons like colds, diarrheas, childbirth and problems of old age—reasons not directly related to their leprosy infection. As with most things in life, familiarity breeds contempt. After one associates with the hospital for a time, one begins to think of the infirmary patients as the unfortunate sick ones and the many other residents of the hospital, in spite of their leprosy, are nothing more than the normal members of the community. To a great extent, most leprosy really has all the earmarks of being an unfortunate circumstance rather than an illness.

It is perhaps fortunate that this disease is not quick to occur. It is a slow chronic illness. Its progress as an infection is measured by the year. The first diagnosis on a patient is often made because of a patch of skin that looks and feels different—not sore but not normal. The person has been aware of the problem for some time and has watched it for at least a year, often much longer, while it very slowly, almost imperceptibly becomes more and more evident. Finally, usually with hesitant doubt, it is decided that help is needed. Leprosy progresses so slowly that it never really becomes a problem until it is an undeniable problem.

While the slow progression of leprosy may be a blessing in one sense, in another sense that slowness is a curse. As one might expect, treatment will not reverse this slow process overnight. Leprosy is long in the course of conquest, firm in its hold and slow to surrender. The time that was not important as the disease slowly progressed now becomes a problem as one, finally having acknowledged its presence, wants it to depart rapidly.

Patience becomes the saving grace of the patients. Aside from a few designated daily chores assigned to some by the administration, the majority of patients spend a good portion of each day in contemplating the illness which controls their life in much the same manner that one refers to the slow, casual, nothing-to-do passage of time as "contemplating one's navel." At best the patient must anticipate years of daily dependence on the science of medicine. Each day, day after day, a bit of time is spent going through the ceremony of the medical ritual. In spite of the dedication that is applied to the routine, the best that the medical community can offer is progress that is so imperceptible that any sense of improvement is based on faith and the word of the doctor.

The patient, not having the training to appreciate the slow certainty of the cure, may be forgiven for an occasional lapse of faith. When this occurs, the patient fills this void by looking to the church for relief from this disease that they often see as a form of punishment for sins that they can't recall having committed. The priest is often more a part of the patient's life than is the physician. When the priest isn't looking, the local faith healer frequently assumes a role, offering hope through the supernatural. Leprosy hospitals see much of this search for relief through the spiritual world.

Faith provides the strength that allows the leprosy patient to survive each long day of many, many days. He places that faith in the three forces that he sees as offering hope for relief from his infirmity: medicine, church and the old spirits. It is often said that there are no atheists on a battlefield. The same can be said for the leprosy community. It was this faith of the leper that in days of old made kings and even bishops and popes, in search of certain admission to heaven, wash the feet of the lepers. I can vouch for the fact that those of us who have lived with these people become infected, not with their disease, but certainly with an appreciation of their fervor.

On occasion the manifestation of the faith of a leprosy patient provides a story unusual enough to bear repeating. Dalmacia was such a patient. She was one of those people that I knew only as a bed patient. In fact I must admit that I never heard her full name and I never thought of inquiring. This is not unusual inside of a leprosarium. Family names are frequently changed or hidden to cover the supposed disgrace that the disease brings on the family. Dalmacia is how I knew her, and Dalmacia is how I will always remember her. She was one of those unfortunate few bedridden people in the Eversley Childs Sanitarium. Even more than this, Dalmacia was an occupant of the "dying bed" for all of the three years that I knew her.

The dying bed was always in a corner, near a window through which the morning sun shone and the cool evening breezes came. It was out of the busy area of the infirmary, but not hidden out of sight. It is almost certain that the good nuns had a hand in the selection of this prime location for the final days. While the corner bed was certainly indicative of a poor medical status, the patient who was assigned to the bed never seemed to accept it as an act of condemnation nor to resent the assignment. The patient's location became a challenge to improve rather than resign to the illness. The corner bed signified special privilege, perhaps better said, special attention.

Dalmacia was unique. Her infection was not at all what one would expect from the textbook. She had no sores; her entire body was sore. In spite of the nun's constant attention and personal, cajoling feeding, Dalmacia wasted away. She was not much more than her skin over bone. The long period of inactivity had atrophied her muscles, leaving her lying in an almost constant fetal position. The sound of that statement rings of horror, but if there was horror, it certainly was not evident when you were in her presence. The skin over her face was smooth, and while there appeared to

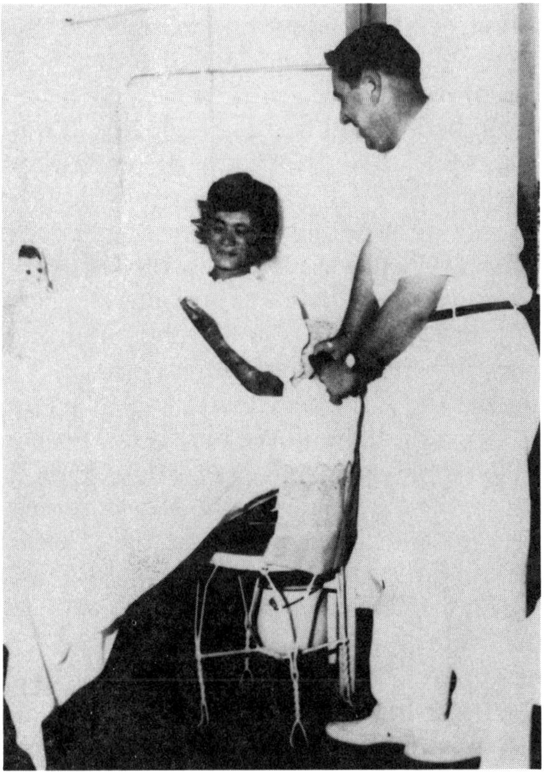

Dalmacia was one of those patients that I knew only as a bed patient—an occupant of the "dying bed" for all of the three years that I knew her.

be little flesh beneath the skin, her face had the smooth taut attraction of that of a woman who starves herself for beauty. Beyond the physical attraction, Dalmacia had an inner beauty that glowed. That beauty blinded the viewer to her illness.

The person inside of Dalmacia's body was unaffected by leprosy. It was only that her body simply refused to respond to any kind of treatment that was offered to her, and many kinds were tried. It was obvious that she no longer had faith in her medicine. Her total faith, and there was much of that, resided in the church, but not in the hope of a cure. Dalmacia had resigned herself to her fate. She was seeking comfort.

She laughed when I first talked to her. It was the musical sound of pleasure. I forget what remark caused it. It doesn't really matter. Laughter from this object, attempting to hide herself by huddling under the dazzling white sheets of the infirmary bed, was absolutely the last thing to be expected. Her attempt to hide was not out of fear or shame. It was the normal reticence of the Philippine woman, an attempt to avoid being the center of attention.

Dalmacia and I became friends. Each day I tried to take a few moments to stop and see her, to talk with her. It became a daily challenge to make her laugh again. Some days it was easy; some days even talking was a problem for her. These visits became a part of my routine. They continued month after month. She appeared to enjoy them as much as I did. It became obvious that she was looking forward to my visits. The nun helped her to sit up for me and to comb and ready herself for my visit. She no longer appeared to be losing the battle of her health and slowly she even began to show signs of improvement. Dalmacia not only sat up in the bed, eventually she hung her legs over the edge of the bed, and finally one day she surprised me by being seated in a chair next to the bed when I arrived.

These visits were good for all of the other women in that ward as well as for Dalmacia. They were all participating in the discourse. They helped Dalmacia ready herself before I arrived and talked with her about my visit after I left. Sometimes, on the occasion of my visits, the healthier girls or children and friends from outside of the infirmary would put on short programs of entertainment in the center of the ward and between the beds.

On that day that Dalmacia got out of her bed, I knew there was something special afoot as I approached the infirmary. Every patient along my route knew what was ahead of me and everyone smiled knowingly at me as I said hello in passing. The ward was unusually quiet as I entered and then I saw her sitting in the chair next to her bed, her lustrous black hair spilling over the white sheet in which she was wrapped. Everyone in the ward was looking at her and she was smiling from ear to ear. It was a most memorable occasion, not just for her, but for all of us who were sharing in her triumph. The entire ward was indulging in an orgy of good feeling. When the cauldron of human emotion finally calmed down, we had a program of Philippine songs and dances. Sister Benigna, the nun in charge of the female infirmary, beamed. She had spent much time preparing for this occasion. She had engineered it.

The happiness of that visit was tempered for me by the knowledge that I would soon be leaving the Philippines. I was being recalled to my laboratory in the United States. The nun and I both knew, but we didn't tell Dalmacia then. We had time. Over the next several months the nun and I slowly broke the word that my visits would be ending soon and when the time finally arrived, Dalmacia seemed to be well adjusted to the idea of my leaving.

On the occasion of my last visit to the infirmary. Dalmacia was again in ecstasy. She had another surprise for me. She was seated in a wheelchair, waiting for me outside, on the flower-studded veranda of the infirmary. As I came up the outside stairs to the building, she wheeled herself toward me and met me at the top of the stairs with the biggest grin that she had ever shown. I didn't have to act; this was a surprise and I showed it. The entire patient group, who had shared in her secret practice sessions, laughed joyfully. They could see in my surprise that they had kept the secret well.

I said good-bye and placed a gift rosary around her neck. Dalmacia and I sat side by side and even touched hands occasionally during the usual program of Filipiniana. This is the ultimate feeling of joyful sorrow.

About three months later, in my office at Johns Hopkins University in Baltimore, I received a letter from Sister Benigna. She wrote to tell me that Dalmacia had told her that she had dreamed that I had been killed in an airplane accident on my way home. It seems that I came to see her in her dream and she saw and spoke with me. According to her dream, I was in heaven and she told the nun that I had talked to her and that I had asked her to join me there.

All this I had already known sometime before the nun's letter arrived. About a month earlier I had gotten a cable from a colleague saying that Dalmacia thought that I had died and that she was planning to join me in heaven. I sent a return cable to Dalmacia assuring her that I was alive and that a letter from me would follow. I wrote to her immediately.

When this letter from the nun arrived, I thought that it was the assurance for which I was waiting. However, after telling me what I already knew, the nun went on to say that Dalmacia had enjoyed the letter that I had sent to her, but she told them she knew that the staff was trying to fool her. She thanked them for their concern. She knew their intentions were good, but last night she had again dreamed that I was calling her. This time she told them that she had promised me in her dream that she would join me. In spite of the fact that she appeared to be physically well, Dalmacia died during the night.

It was on that first Christmas day after my return to the Philippines that I visited her gravesite on a slight rise overlooking the blue channel of water that separates this island from its neighbor. It is behind the leprosarium—a silent, lonely place, one of a very few where one can be alone on a very crowded tropical island. I was uncertain and disturbed. The scientist in me spoke aloud to no one in particular, wondering how Dalmacia's leprosy could possibly have gotten so much better over such a long period of time while she was still using a drug that had previously been failing for such a long time. The person inside of me quietly wondered if the capacity to achieve the kind of strength that Dalmacia had shown was a form of compensation for leprosy. Is it really possible that the rigors of bearing the burden of leprosy allow one to acquire a greater faith, to see things to which the rest of us are blind?

In the midst of my troubled reverie, I became aware that the bell in the old chapel in the leprosarium behind me was calling the patients to the Christmas service. The peal of the bell broke the stillness and brought the old song to mind: "I heard the bells on Christmas day, the old familiar carols play . . . " However, everyone knows that the bell at Eversley can not sing. It goes clink, clank, clink, clunk. It has no voice for singing. Yet as it began to intrude into my thoughts, I found that I was mouthing words to its beat and, in my mind's eye, the little bell slowly changed its voice, finally rivaling the grand bell of a great cathedral as I slowly repeated after it . . . cling, clang, cling, clunk . . . DING, DONG, DING, DONG . . . BONG, BONG, BONG, BONG . . . MER-REE CHRISTMAS . . . DAL-MAH-SEE-YAH . . . I heard it long after the chapel bell ceased tolling. I knew that the answer to my dilemma lay in what she believed and how strongly she believed it. She became well as a matter of faith.

Somehow just realizing that I had found some sort of rationalization to my doubt did not change my mood. I slowly turned and walked back toward the colony. Suddenly I was awakened from my trance by the sound of young voices. The children from the leprosarium, and there were many, surrounded me. They were clapping sleighbells made from bottle caps loosely nailed onto one end of foot-long pieces of wood, much like the warning

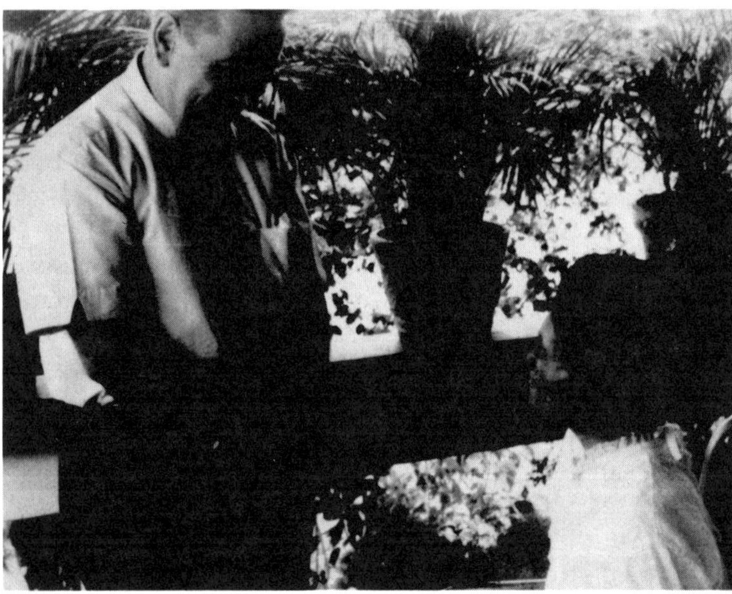

Dalmacia was seated in a wheelchair, waiting for me outside, on the flower-studded veranda of the infirmary. Today, unlike the practice for centuries past, her kind of leprosy no longer achieves the special attention of the dying bed.

clappers of the medieval leper. Children rarely show signs of the disease, and it is never seen in the very young, so they need to warn no one of their presence; they were using their clappers as bells to accompany their singing of "Jingle Bells."

They followed me into the hospital grounds, jumping, running, skipping and singing loudly, "Hinkle bells, hinkle bells . . . Merry Christmas, *Dooktor*. Do you have a *cinco*?" A *cinco* is a five-*centavo* coin worth about one fourth of a U.S. penny. They followed me, laughing, singing and joyously begging a pittance. Our little gathering went past the chapel, where the service had just finished. Smiling patients were leaving and laughing and chattering away without evidence that they had any care in the world. As I passed them they would laugh at my noisy little gathering and say, "Good morning, *Dooktor*, Merry Christmas."

Suddenly I felt better also, and I realized that I had gone from darkness into sunlight within the two hundred yards between the grave of Dalmacia and the chapel. There the sky had matched my somber mood and here the sun shone brightly. The slender palm trees were now outlined against a deep blue sky and the sea below sparkled with an ever-changing pattern of bright specks of light. These things had really been the same just a few minutes ago, but I had not been seeing them. That difference in brightness and mood was not real. It was not the world that had changed in this short span; it was me. It was what I wanted to believe. It was a matter of faith. Even the sound of the bell had been a matter of faith. Faith needs no scientific explanation. It only needs to be there. That was the message of this day. The Filipino says *Malagayong Pasko*. We say Merry Christmas. Doesn't it seem strange that it means the same thing no matter how you say it. It is merely a matter of faith.

Less than two years later the scientists at Eversley

Childs cooperated in the development of a drug that would have corrected Dalmacia's infirmity. Today, unlike the practice for centuries past, her kind of leprosy no longer achieves the special attention of the dying bed.

Four

At Home and Play: Another Culture

In the late summer of 1961, Dr. James Angus Doull, then the medical director of the Leonard Wood Memorial Foundation, asked me if I could design a small fundamental laboratory suitable for construction in the tropics and adequate for the purpose of conducting good basic scientific work on leprosy. It was a Friday evening and that fact only becomes important and memorable because of the timing. Doull was just returning home from a visit to India and the Philippines. On the way home, he telephoned me at my home in Baltimore, from Cleveland, where he was visiting friends. He called because he wanted me to think about the problem over the weekend. He wasn't sure whether the new lab would be in India or the Philippines, but he felt that it should be at a site where the study materials were most available, inside of a leprosy hospital.

I was honored, pleased and excited. I answered immediately, "I most certainly can. When do you want the plans?"

He responded, "I would like to see an outline of your working plans Monday morning in my office in Washington." He didn't ask if that was possible. He simply said, " . . . Monday morning."

Somehow, I'll never tell you how, but I arrived in his office two days later, Monday morning, with a set of drawings that, with little or no changes from the original, later became the Leonard Wood Memorial—Eversley Childs laboratory for leprosy research. I honestly believe that if I had been given more time to think about the problem, that spontaneous efficiency would not have occurred. Over the years, the plans have been unbelievably effective in practical use.

I first arrived in Cebu in October of 1962 and the laboratory was already under construction. Dr. Doull had initiated the work himself during an earlier visit that he made in the summer of 1962. He had asked me to accompany him on that visit. I begged off on that occasion to attend to the details that were required for my emigration to Cebu with my wife and a seven-year-old daughter.

I had much to do before I could leave home. There remained a matter of my continued obligations to the research program of Dr. John Hanks. He was my colleague in the Leonard Wood Memorial and my immediate superior in the leprosy research being conducted in the laboratory at Johns Hopkins University. I also had to plan and order all laboratory equipment and supplies for Cebu and arrange for their shipment to the new laboratory. I was also still designing the interior fixtures of the lab: cabinets, workbenches and tables. These were to be made, in place, in Cebu by native Philippine carpenters. There were electric lines and lighting, water lines and sinks to plan.

Just as a minor task, it was also necessary to put my personal affairs in order for an extended stay in the Philippines. The length of that stay was never agreed upon. Dr. Doull merely suggested, "The usual tour of duty for assignments like this is five years. We'll cross that bridge when we come to it." The uncertainty of that time agreement haunted me later. However, the year of preparation before leaving the U.S. was so demanding that I never had time to think about something that was as unimportant as when I would be coming home again.

It appears that I survived that year of preparation, but when I look back over those days, I can't imagine how. The entire year was a process of close timing and I mean close. The narrow margins and deadlines followed me right down to the last minute before leaving. The passports for me and my family reached us at out hotel in the hour before we boarded the ship in New York harbor.

The passports with proper visas were sent from Washington, D.C. to our hotel in New York by messenger from Dr. Doull. The delay was caused by Dr. Doull's insistence that I needed a tax-exempt Philippine visa. These were hard to acquire. We had been in contact with the Philippine Embassy in Washington all summer without final approval. Dr. Doull was insistent. He wanted to establish the precedent for anyone in the foundation who might follow me to Cebu. We still had not been granted our visas by September, and by that time, all of our family furniture had been placed in storage. We were no longer living in our home in Baltimore. Finally, Dr. Doull instructed me to leave Baltimore on schedule without our passports. He promised that he would see that I had them in time to leave the country. I was ready for a mental breakdown by the time those travel requirements were in my hands. I have never been good at last-minute planning. Dr. Doull was a master. He never did learn that while he had succeeded in getting me a visa that said "Tax Exempt," I never really was. Is anyone, anywhere ever really "tax exempt"?

Somehow we managed to keep going in spite of a constant sour stomach. We left our home in early September 1962 for a strange place and an unbelievable challenge. We left New York on the ship *Bremen* bound for London where, while en route to Cebu, I would be attending a meeting of the International Leprosy Association. Those five days on shipboard were the treatment that was necessary to relieve the tensions of the last year. I didn't realize it then, but they were the last five successive days of just plain relaxation that I can recall for the rest of my professional life. Dr. Doull knew what I was facing—he had prescribed this trip.

After the meeting, we flew from London to the Philippines. A crash landing in Bombay brought me face to face with the fact that prayer would most likely become an important part of my daily existence. A broken panel light indicated that the nosewheel of the Boeing 707 did not drop into position for the landing. The pilot, uncertain whether the failure was just the pilot light or in reality the nosewheel, made a series of low level passes over Bombay airport in the dark hours before dawn. The ground crew, using a searchlight to light up the underbelly of the plane as it passed rapidly over their heads, failed to determine the status of the wheel.

The aerial maneuvers seemed to continue forever. For some reason the air conditioning in the 707 was not working during these aerobic manipulations, and the heat inside of the plane became unbearable. Finally, with a great deal of uncertainty, part of which he expressed to the passengers, the pilot brought the plane down onto the runway with a resounding thump to free the wheel if possible. The thump was followed by a long, long trip down the runway with everyone, in crash position, anticipating the moment when the nose came down. The eventual contact of the nosewheel on the runway was solid, and the realization that all was well brought a spontaneous round of applause from a planeload of very nervous passengers. The applause was followed by an unbelievable silence during which nearly every passenger on the plane suddenly became ill. The line of fire and emergency equipment that could be seen returning up the runway as we disembarked did not help to do anything except to confirm that our prayers had been necessary and apparently effective.

The landing in Bombay signaled that our old life was now behind us; our next stop in Calcutta confirmed that our new life had begun. I had to stop in Calcutta to carry some messages to several of my Johns Hopkins colleagues who were conducting public health studies in India. I remained only one week, but the impossible human existence that we saw during that week became very important as a buffer to any possible culture shock that might await us in the Philippines. Calcutta prepared us for Manila and Manila for Cebu. In the long run, the final unbelievable isolation of Cebu from the rest of the world became the only hardship that we had to overcome. That isolation actually became a blessing when it came time to face the leprosy problem at its source.

So, now to build a laboratory. I arrived in October. The contractor had started in June and he promised that I would have a laboratory before the spring of 1963, in about four more months. He was wrong. We finally dedicated the laboratory in February of 1964, one year, four and one-half months after my arrival on Cebu. To relate all of the problems of those many months would be beating a dead horse, but some of the tales do bear repeating in the sense that they are indeed some of the more colorful of the memories that became "Blossoms from the Kalatuchi Tree."

I had never really built anything bigger than a sandcastle or a Boy Scout lean-to before this journey. That fact was not important. Like most young folk with a few courses in mechanical drawing, I felt that I could draw plans for anything that I could dream about, and if I could draw them, I could build them. The thought of overseeing the construction of those plans never entered my mind.

If Dr. Doull had remained on the scene, I would have felt more secure, but Dr. Doull succumbed to a terminal illness shortly after I commenced my duties in Cebu. Not only did I lose a good friend and medical director, but unbelievable indecision within the Leonard Wood Memorial Foundation after his death caused the office of medical director to remain empty during the entire period of laboratory construction. Not only was the office to which I looked for advice and counsel empty, but the people in the administration of the foundation and all of its U.S. employees seemed to have forgotten that there was a program in Cebu. I received almost no official mail for something in the order of one year, and most of my urgent pleas home went unanswered.

I was forced to rely on my own resources to build my dream, and when I say resources, I do mean resources. At one time, due to tardy reimbursement of expenses from the home office, I had more than five thousand dollars of my own funds in the laboratory construction. This lack of communication complicated many of my problems. I had a shipment of laboratory equipment and supplies on a boat somewhere between New York and Manila. I got no response to my repeated letters begging someone, anyone to please clarify the status of that shipment. I needed desperately to know if the laboratory items would arrive before or after I had a laboratory to store them. I never did find out until they arrived fortunately after the laboratory was ready to receive them.

Of more immediate concern, was a shipment of personal clothing, bedding, toiletries and household items. My wife and I had carefully crated and shipped these things to Cebu several months before we left home in the hope that they would arrive in the Philippines about the same time that we did. When I queried the whereabouts of this crate shortly after our arrival in Cebu, I was told that it had been lost somewhere in the half of the world through which it had to travel to reach us, but that I should not worry, since they had already put a tracer on it. Two months later, just one week before Christmas 1962 I got a message from the shipping agents in Manila that my crate had been burned in a recent large fire on the docks in Manila.

It is not completely true that I had no correspondence with the foundation in that first year. I did receive a few letters from the adminstration in America, but since there was no person there who was familiar with my project, I got no intelligent answers. I remember only one of the return messages. I probably will never forget it. It was the epitome of what is called "gobbledygook." In response to a plea that I made to the home office that I should be allowed to make a quick trip home to straighten out a number of problems, I received a call stating only, "Your request to travel denied (stop) Sorry (stop) Your return would be only one side of the story." I have thought of that message often and questioned it later. No one seems to remember it but me. My immediate request for clarification of the message was never answered.

In spite of the travel denial, I thought seriously of returning home anyway at my own expense to see just what was happening back there and how it was going to affect my work in Cebu. However, I could barely afford a single fare on my own, and I was too new to the territory to trust leaving my wife and daughter alone in Cebu. Up until that time, Cebu was still an uncertain and apparently hostile environment to me.

I suppose in retrospect, everyone experiences some period in their life that later can be seen as the low point of their existence. My first three months in Cebu must be considered as a good candidate for that spot in my life. However, it is often said that "it is always darkest before the dawn." On the Friday before Christmas 1962, in true keeping with that thought, a big flat-body truck pulled up before our house and delivered one huge crate filled with household items, clothing, toys and marvelous memories of home. It seems that our personal belongings had not burned. The crate had been put on board an interisland ship for transit to Cebu just before the pier in Manila caught fire. The darkest period in our life also happened to include the most wonderful Christmas ever. One can live for a while out of suitcases, but really not for too long.

New Year's Eve before 1963 was an education. It was our introduction to the kind of revelry that still existed on this, one of the last outposts of old-style colonial Asian existence. I say "colonial" because that characteristic was very evident in the evening cocktail affairs in the country club and in the private parties at the homes of the foreign residents. This atmosphere of full dress, party games and crystal martini glasses was markedly different from the atmosphere in the city neighborhoods, around the harbor and out into the countryside. The Chinese influence dominated the evening in these places, and to the Chinese a New Year celebration requires noise.

Fireworks of all kinds were the order of the night. Rockets began to fill the skies starting before midnight and ending before dawn. I do mean that rockets filled the skies. The din was continuous for several hours. The constant roar of explosives was so unbelievable to me that I recorded thirty minutes of it. Taken out of context, the recording was only a very dull constant cacophony of sound that proved worthless. One of the more memorable incidents of that first Cebu New Year occurred about thirty minutes after midnight when an enormous blast rattled our window louvres and almost destroyed our eardrums. Someone in the party next door had set off dynamite—dynamite mind you, not a firecracker—in his neighbor's driveway. Next morning it was discovered that the explosion had shattered the concrete driveway and broken a number of windows. Happy New Year 1963!

I never thought it possible, but there actually did come a day when I moved into the new laboratory. It was not yet totally completed, but I managed to find workspace in a corner of the building, away from the final effort of the contractor. Up until then I had been conducting haphazard microbiology in two small areas that I managed to confiscate in the old clinical facilities of the foundation. One of the temporary work areas was at the Cebu Skin Clinic in the city of Cebu, and the other was at the sanitarium in a building near the new construction.

The primitive nature of these facilities made me feel like one of the early pioneers in the science of microbiology. In both places the work areas were in the open-sided tropical shelters that are common to the Philippines. They have louvered side openings in place of windows. The soft breezes through the open louvres made for pleasant working conditions in this hot climate, but I often wondered if Louis Pasteur had to cope with flies walking across his microscope stage. I did have a pressure cooker to sterilize my test tubes but I had no incubator for my early culture trials. I am not too sure that an incubator was necessary in this tropical climate.

It was during this period in my life that I became familiar with the reality of Murphy's law: "If anything can go wrong, it will." The contractor had given fate every opportunity to demonstrate the value of the law. The greatest of these problems occurred shortly after my arrival in Cebu. The contractor, in response to my query, informed me that the rear center door from the basement would come out of the building in the air, roughly twenty feet above the ground. This was true not only for the rear door, but also for the entire rear of the building which was supported by square concrete pillars rising out of the side of the hill.

The contractor informed me that he had made this change, prior to my arrival, on the orders of my Philippine colleagues. Apparently, they had not cared for my drawings showing a ground level entrance in the front. They wanted the building to have a more impressive facade. The contractor was asked to raise the first floor a full half story above the ground level and install a set of terrazzo tile stairs leading up to the front entrance of the building. Everyone seems to have forgotten that if the front is raised, the back also goes up. Neither Dr. Doull nor I was informed of this change. It only became obvious to me later when I noticed that while the front looked impressive, the rear looked uncertain. By the time the foundation problem was disclosed, Dr. Doull was no longer available to help me with the correction.

A retaining wall was obviously required to support the rear of the building. Before it was completed, this retaining wall consumed almost as much concrete as the entire laboratory which, incidentally, was built entirely of reinforced concrete. The base of the wall when it was finished rested on a slab of concrete about fifty feet long, one yard deep by three yards wide. The wall was erected on top of this slab along the edge away from the building. In this way, the weight of the building was on the rear of the slab and prevented the wall from tilting away from the building. The wall was fifty feet long, twenty feet high, one yard wide at the bottom and narrowed to about one foot wide at the top. All of this concrete was mixed in a small gasoline motor mixer at the site. The sand, stones and cement were put into the mixer by hand, by the shovelful.

As could be anticipated following Murphy's law, there was a strike in the local cement plant at this time. The law of supply and demand made the price of cement exorbitant. Cement was available by "special arrangement" only. Special arrangement means "available with political assistance" Guess what that means.

Outside of the building, the wall was the major problem. Inside of the building, the big problem was the pipes: water lines, gas lines, electrical conduit. These were all assembled on top of the network of reinforcing rods inside of the forms for the cement of the concrete main floor. When all pipes and rods were in place, a mass of concrete about six inches thick was poured over, around and under these service pipes.

It sounds permanent and it was, but in a chat with the contractor, I discovered that the cement had been poured before the pipes had been tested for leaks. I was willing to take a chance on the water pipes, but I admitted to cowardice when it came to using untested gas lines buried in concrete. I finally did test the embedded lines using compressed air and they appeared to be without leaks.

These positive results made me a bit braver. However, my compressed air test still showed a slight drop in pressure that probably was due to temperature changes, but I wasn't sure. I woke up at night visualizing an explosion resulting from a slow leak that could form gas pockets within the concrete mass. To satisfy this concern, I hooked the embedded gas line to the water pump and I kept water under pressure in the system for several days. Fortunately, we never saw any wet spots in the concrete. That water test procedure may have alleviated my concern for a gas leak, but the water, once in the gas line, was not so easy to remove. For some months after we started using the gas line, an occasional Bunsen burner would sputter and a bit of water would squirt out through the flame.

The cement-encased electrical conduits were successfully threaded with the proper service lines, and all went well except for moderate grounding of some of the lighting circuits. I suspected that some of the wiring lost a bit of insulation here and there by being drawn too forcefully into the tubing. This problem never became serious, and any immediate correction to the wiring in the conduits was not worth the effort. It is true that the fluorescent lights in the basement glowed softly during the night even when the switches were turned off. This eerie glow gave additional impetus to the later discovery that the laboratory was haunted. In the years that followed, I managed to bypass the shorted electric lines with new lines strung outside of the conduits.

There were other events of interest during this period of construction. Only one was significant enough to merit description as a memoir "blossom" in itself. Two closets were included in the plans for the basement kitchen and prep room. In lab terms, a kitchen is the place where the glassware is washed, sterilized and stored. These closets were each to be four feet wide and two feet deep with doors thirty inches wide. Of course, on completion I found that the closet doors were made to open inward. I got angry and objected to what I called "lack of brains." In return, I was criticized sharply for not making it perfectly clear on the plans that I wanted the closet doors to open outward.

Another incident deserves to be assigned a value of only half of a "blossom." That incident is about the dumbwaiter that served to carry glassware and supplies between the kitchen in the basement and the main laboratory on the floor above. In view of my earlier failure to specify which way the closet doors should open, I went into great detail to stress the necessity for an adequate cable to hold the dumbwaiter. I wanted to be sure that the contractor did not use cord string to fasten the dumbwaiter through the overhead pulley that was fastened to a beam under the roof. He did use a good adequate cable, but I did not foresee that he would use only a single bent nail to hold the upper pulley to the beam under the roof. That nail pulled out one day when the tray, filled with glassware, reached the upper pulley. I was later proudly informed that the cable did not break.

It was during this period in my life that I coined the motto, "A catastrophe a day makes for a better flavor to my evening nip of Scotch." There was always a "belt o' Scotch" sitting on the bar for me when I came home for dinner. My wife allowed me time to savor my wee nip, then allowed me a bit more time to retire to my bedroom. There I cried, composed myself and returned to dinner.

My life in Cebu wasn't only devoted to the laboratory. Life went on at home also. Among other things, we managed to meet and adopt Tony Teneriffe. He was a kindly, middle-aged man who came door to door selling seashells. At first he came to our house one day a week, and each time we bought a few, so he started to come two days a week, three days a week and so on. Tony finally became a daily visitor. We have a very large collection of shells.

One day Tony's wife came instead of Tony, and she informed us that Tony was very ill in the local hospital. If she could not get some money for his medicine, Tony was going to die. By this time we had Tony figured as being a bit of a schemer and a bit short of truthful. I called the hospital and was told that the story was indeed true. It seems that in this part of the world, medicine is a marketable commodity. Those who can afford it can get it; those who can't afford it must trust in fate. Tony was in the hands of fate. I was horrified, but I recognized this as another one of those differences in culture. I informed the hospital that I would pay for Tony's medication. My word was enough, he was given the medicine; he survived; I never got charged for the medicine. I was told that they could not charge me because I was dedicating my life to help the Philippine people. That is the problem of the Third World, it always needs a middle man to help itself.

Tony, the "shell man," taught me much about the anomalies of life in strange cultures. I could understand not being charged for the medicine, and I was most grateful. That act was in keeping with the gracious character of these people, but Tony was on the other side of the coin. I did not anticipate that since I had saved Tony's life, he now belonged to me. At least that was Tony's understanding as to how the local culture functioned. He was now at my call, or so he said. I also had to accept the responsibility of being available to ease any further financial emergencies in the Teneriffe family. That was a situation that I soon informed Tony was not to my liking, but his ingenuity knew no boundaries. Since I would not provide total support to the Tenneriffe family, Tony did the next best thing. He offered to sell members of his family to me from time to time at bargain prices.

The unwillingness of the Philippine physicians to charge me for any personal medical problems was one of the many positive factors of our life in Cebu. One time my wife had emergency surgery for a kidney stone. This required several weeks of hospitalization. Another time, I was hospitalized for one month with two fractured vertebrae. On both occasions neither the doctors nor the hospitals would accept any money from me. Their attention to our well-being in both situations was overwhelming.

The medical emergency for Mrs. Reich occurred while we were attending a local movie. She made it home from the theater, but she was not feeling well at all. Shortly after our arrival home, the pain became unbearable and I immediately drove her in to the nearest hospital. Here they surgically relieved a blocked ureter which had been causing a severe kidney problem. I was informed that it would be necessary for me to be present in the surgery during the operation. That is a common procedure here. It is intended to assure the family that the surgeon is doing his best for the patient. It is sort of an Oriental version of malpractice insurance.

Her stay in Perpetual Succor Hospital was accompanied by unbelievable attention on the part of the staff. Her every whim was their command. She was given one of the best rooms in the hospital. It had a refrigerator that was working and made ice cubes. Ice cubes go well with Scotch, and the ice cubes were the lure that led to our meeting with Father Nolan. The good father was a young priest with a broad brogue that left little doubt as to his ancestry. He was a patient at the time and had the room across the corridor, but the refrigerator in that room was not working.

Father Shawn Nolan had a parish on Camiguin, a small island just off the coast of Mindanao. He had been bitten by a rabid dog which is far too common a problem in the Philippines. At that time, in this place, the treatment for rabies was a series of twenty-four injections. These were not available in his little island parish, and so he came to Cebu to stay until his series was completed. He was boarded in this church-sponsored hospital for his comfort and for the doctor's convenience. This was his first trip away from his parish in over three years, and he was relishing this rabies cure.

On occasion, I would join him in sipping on an ice cube or two and listen to the tales of life on his island. I still remember his story about one of the young boxers in the youth program that he sponsored. The young fellow made cement building blocks for a living. His professional name as a boxer was "The Hollow Block Kid."

Nolan's stories were told in Irish brogue so thick that it was almost a foreign language to my Pennsylvania German ears. How does one interpret, "Ahh yes, you should taste the rrrroooooommm ooomlet that me cooook makes?" After I got past the rolling rs, I did manage to understand that his Filipino cook made a good rum omelet. He not only told me about it, but during his last few days in the hospital, he cabled his cook to come to Cebu to accompany him back to Camiguin. While the cook was in Cebu, Father Nolan had him prepare the famous omelet for Val and me. It was then that I discovered that when Father Nolan said rrrroooooommm, he really meant rum. Boy did he mean rum!

My stay in Cebu Doctor's Hospital came considerably later in my career when I was almost constantly commuting between Baltimore and Cebu. The hospitalization was the result of two broken vertebrae. It was without the pleasure of Father Nolan's wit and support, but all of my medical attention was given graciously, attentively and without charge.

I had been staying in the Cebu Plaza Hotel at the time of the medical misadventure. At three I was, as usual, wide awake and preparing to leave for the airport to catch a plane out of Cebu. While doing some last-minute writing at the desk, I noticed a rather large cockroach on the ceiling above me. The roach is a fact of life in Cebu and one eventually learns to disregard the presence of the noble beast. On finishing my writing, I got up abruptly from the desk chair to go to the bathroom. By now the cockroach had moved and was halfway down on the wall next to the desk and was between me and the bathroom door. My abrupt movement startled her into a mad rush for the floor. In turn, this startled me into a step backward, which in turn caused me to flip backward over the desk chair. I landed on my "tushi" and found that I couldn't get back up.

I managed to drag myself to the door where I slipped the chain and then back to the nightstand where I got the telephone and called the desk to send help. For one brief moment during all of this dragging across the floor, my roach friend had the temerity to walk across the floor in front of me and stop. She wiggled her long antennae in my direction as if she was trying to communicate. I reached for a folded newspaper and eyed her staring back at me within easy swatting distance. The temptation was very great, but I resisted it; instead I merely tapped the paper in front of her, sending her scurrying under the wall to what I like to think was her husband and kids. One of my major accomplishments in life has been the ability to determine the sex of a cockroach at a glance. The female is much, much larger than the male. He's about half the size of my thumbnail. She's as large as my thumb.

Help and an ambulance soon arrived and I was taken to the hospital where X rays revealed the painful truth of the cracked bones. Fortunately, the nature of the problem required nothing more than an extended bed rest until the bones healed enough to allow me to sit and stand up again. Pain alone was to be the determining factor in the duration of my cure. For at least two weeks, I was convinced that I would never ever sit up again. When sitting became possible it took another week during which I thought that I most likely will never be able to walk again. Finally, thirty days after my encounter with the skittish roach, the pain was down to a level that I could tolerate it enough to finally leave the hospital on crutches. I went from the hospital in Cebu to the airport in Reading, Pennsylvania, nonstop.

The physical pain of the broken back was the least of

my worries. Try to explain to people that you broke your back at three A.M. in a hotel because you were scared by a cockroach. My Filipino colleagues all thought that explanation was hilarious. They would whoop, wink, elbow each others ribs and say, "They must have been beautiful cockroaches!"

From closet doors to cockroaches, from Calcutta to Cebu, from retaining walls to omelets, and from the country club to life in a leprosarium, the unchanging seasons of the tropics went on day after day. There were times when I stepped out of the house in the morning and faced the rising sun with a prayer for just one lungful of air so cold that I could see my breath. I think that I'll nevermore want to live in a land without at least a mild form of winter. My life has taught me that without winter, there is no spring. Just as winter brings the spring, so too did the harsh problems of my entry into life in Cebu bring me a greater sense of the beauty of this "Land of the Morning Sun."

I learned to understand and admire the Kalatuchi tree. In a land without seasons there is still a time in the year when it loses its leaves and rests for a while. It blooms again later in full scented beauty. It has found a way to remain true to its own nature in spite of the events around it. This process is essential to all living things that wish to pursue a useful life in a strange world, perhaps even in their own.

Five

The Spirit of the Tree: A Lady Ghost

The opportunity to build a modern medical research laboratory on a tropical island is granted to few people. The opportunity to build that laboratory inside of a leprosarium on a tropical island is sought by few people. To finish that laboratory and to find it both functional and haunted is rare.

Supposedly, it was haunted because the laboratory was built too close to the ghost tree that had stood for generations along the entrance road to the leprosarium. No one mentioned the problem of the tree when the building site was chosen. To have suggested the tree as a possible problem would have been an admission of belief in such acts of nature. Everyone, even those who now stated with certainty that the laboratory was haunted, would have had a great laugh at such a ridiculous statement.

The first hint of unearthly possession occurred during construction of the laboratory. One dark night the night watchman who guarded the materials and supplies on the site was "rudely tossed from the building by a ghost." There was no question in anyone's mind about this. The next morning it was obvious that the poor man had been badly abused, having apparently been thrown two stories to the ground at the rear of the partially completed structure.

Everyone knew and everyone agreed that the lady spirit of the tree had somehow taken offense at the construction that was being done within less than one hundred yards of her ancient shelter in the heights of the old Tipolo tree.

Just to look at the tree was to know that it was something special. It stood beside the road on the way to the circle of administration buildings. On this island, wood is scarce and valuable. There are too few trees even to provide the firewood that is essential for the many cooking fires that are needed to prepare each day's rice and fish. It took a very special kind of immunity to allow a tree to survive and grow to be about 60 feet tall and more than six feet in trunk

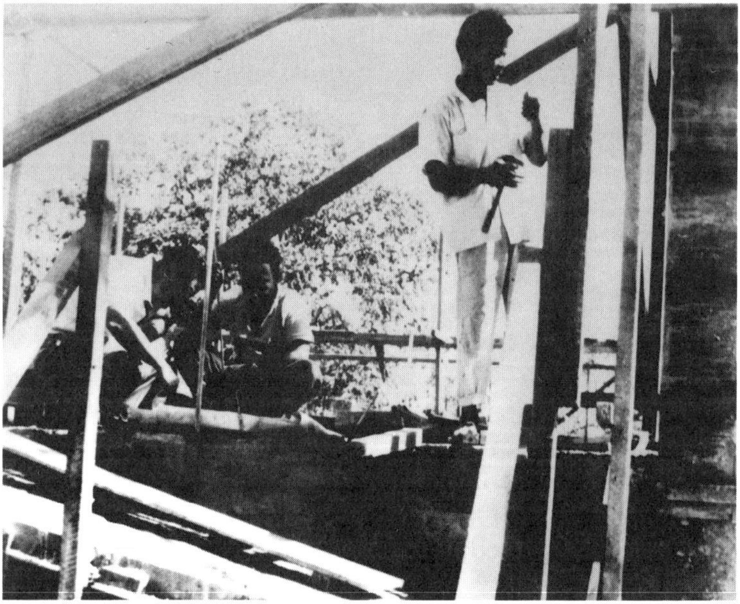

The laboratory, here under construction, was built too close to the ghost tree in background that had stood for generations along the entrance road to the leprosarium.

diameter. The tree's special status was also apparent in the treatment that it was given by the natives. One did not loiter in its shade and everyone moved more quickly past it as the passing day lengthened its shadow. Those of us who were not natives did not fully realize the power that fell within the sphere of its surrounding aura. The laboratory was in that aura.

So the laboratory was haunted at birth. That problem was not significant in the midst of the more pertinent problems that accompanied the act of starting a new research effort in a new facility. To the uninitiated, the haunting had little reality. It was, as everyone agreed, no more than a matter of interest. Life went on and other, more serious problems demanded our attention. However, it soon became clear that meetings were never scheduled for late afternoon in the laboratory. In a climate near the equator, where there is no twilight, where day passes directly into night, this seeming fear of the dark soon became noticeable and demanded an answer.

"Why?"

"Well sir, the laboratory is haunted."

"What can I do about that?"

"The building must be blessed, sir."

"Good grief!"

I had forgotten that; it should have been done. That is the way it is done here. I quickly responded, "I just didn't think, I'm sorry. Will you please make whatever arrangements are necessary to have the laboratory properly blessed? I am sorry that I didn't think about that sooner."

"Yes sir, I will do it, and that is all right, sir."

One fine tropical day all of the employees including the doctors and professional staff formed a circle in the front of the large central room. The three elderly Belgian nuns, who lived in and made the leprosarium really a place of true mercy, joined us. Very old Father McMahon, whose rectory was in the very center of the leprosarium and who had spent a lifetime among these people, conducted the ceremony from a position just inside the door facing the heart of the laboratory.

This was my first house blessing. The circumstances surrounding the haunting and the blessing of the laboratory intrigued my scientist's mind. To me, the ritual assumed all the trappings of a controlled experiment. Would the ghost leave this corner of the domain over which she had exercised power for far longer than any of us, including the aged Father McMahon? When the blessing was completed, I was not sure that I really wanted to lose my ghost. She had become a part of the excitement of my venture into this different way of life.

So the laboratory was blessed and life again assumed its usual abnormal character. For a while all seemed to be as it should be. There was a marked difference in staff behavior. I was even able to hold staff meetings that were not rushed by the fading light of late afternoon. The staff no longer stood up and shuffled as five o'clock approached. They even held social conversation in the library after the meetings were adjourned. However, was it my imagination, or was everyone avoiding the far corner of the building on the side near the ghost tree? I felt that question needed an answer. "Why?" I asked a worker.

"The ghost, sir."

"How could that be, the building has been properly blessed."

"Yes, sir, but Father McMahon is very old sir and he only stood at the one spot during the blessing. His power could not reach that far corner."

"What harm can the ghost do from that far corner?"

"Oh, very much sir, especially after dark."

"But I am often here at night, even after midnight, and I have not been harmed."

"No sir, but we have all confirmed that she is in love with you."

That was enough, the ghost would remain. Fortunately, the men's room was in the safe portion of the building.

Life went on, and we lived with the ghost without any major incident from then on. The knowledge that this spirit power felt kindly toward me and that everyone was awed by this manifestation pleased me. I lived with it and at times flaunted the power. When I walked past the tree, I often looked up into the tree or lingered under its branches. The people nodded knowingly to each other. In this way I shared the power.

One day, one of the nuns told me that everyone in the leprosarium knew that I believed in the ghost.

"Is this true, Doctor?"

I told her that I didn't really know if I believed in the ghost. She told me that she didn't know if she believed either but one night she did have an experience with the ghost.

She told me that about two o'clock one morning, she was returning to her quarters from the infirmary when a piece of wood was thrown at her as she approached the tree. It did not fall from the tree; it was thrown from up in the tree and at her. Thinking that she was being taunted by some mischievous child she called out, "Stop that nonsense, boy." Then another piece of wood nearly hit her as she got under the tree. She got very angry, shouted again and looked up and around with her light to find the culprit. There was nothing there.

"Doctor, I ran and the pieces of wood kept falling behind me, following me even after I was far away from the tree. Mother Superior heard me coming and was waiting as I ran into the residence. She asked me, 'What in the world is wrong, sister?' I told her what had happened and I asked her if she could help me to understand it. Mother said, 'There are many things on this earth that have no explanation.'

"Doctor, I don't know if I believe in the ghost, but I think I do."

It isn't a question of the ghost being real or not real. Everyone in this part of the island knew about this entity who was female and lived in the high branches of the old tree even before their parents' time. Everyone moved around and treated the tree in a manner that took the spirit into consideration. It would have been too obvious to do otherwise. In this sense, the ghost was very real. She was most likely neither all fact nor all fiction. She was certainly a very real part of the local history and custom. If I didn't believe in her, I never openly doubted her.

I profited from this apparent belief. Since it was well known that she favored me, I had a powerful friend in a "high place." The people who knew about these things treated me with the respect due that friendship.

There was only one occasion when I called on that power. There was a perennial conflict with the government representatives in the hospital over water. They felt that they could relieve the institution's chronic water shortage by gaining access to the laboratory's independent water supply. We did provide some water to the infirmaries and for certain critical functions of the institution, but apparently not enough. We couldn't possibly provide enough water to keep the constantly open water taps down in the patient living area satisfied. No one could ever satisfy that demand. We usually gave until it hurt. The argument was not about how much we should supply. It was about how much we could hurt and still survive.

One day the argument became most emotional, and the government officer in charge made a demand that could not be met. He made the mistake of making the demand in the presence of persons of such significance that the demand could not be retracted. To save face, he backed the demand with an order to his maintenance officer to disconnect the laboratory from its water source. First thing in the morning he was to redirect all water from the laboratory into the hospital area. That order was tantamount to a termination of our effort. Reversal of his decision was possible, but only after enough time had lapsed that there was no doubt about the act or about his authority to do it. Then, and only then, would he grant me the privilege of giving me back some of my own water supply. That timing would be very uncertain.

At the time, the laboratory effort was in a critical period that allowed for no long interruption. There was no easy way out of this dilemma. After dinner that evening, I returned to the laboratory to try to modify the experiments to ease the damage from the coming water problem. Much later, after finishing the task, I sat alone in a darkened room in the haunted area of the building. I was smoking a cigarette and contemplating the current sorry state of my existence. Suddenly, I knew what I had to do.

At five minutes before midnight, I walked out of the building, over to the ghost tree, and knelt in the dust in the middle of the road. Within minutes I had attracted a crowd of interested spectators. The patients never seem to sleep—their life is a twenty-four-hour routine. They formed a quiet arc behind me. They remained in the shadows at a distance that they considered to be safe from any possible interference with the lady in the tree.

The grapevine is fast. A few minutes more and Mother Superior was running up the road shouting, "Doctor, Doctor, are you well?"

I said nothing, remaining bowed and silent until she was at my side. Then I said, as calmly as I could, "Yes Mother, I am well, but I have something to do."

She said, "I understand, Doctor," and she quietly stepped back into the dark to join the other silent observers.

After several minutes, I stood up, smiled, and said, "Thank you" aloud to no one in particular. I then walked over to join Mother.

The crowd slowly dispersed and Mother apologized, saying, "At first I thought you were ill." Nothing more was said about my behavior.

Next morning I was told that the government officer had left the island on the first flight out that morning. He had gone to Manila. He did not return to Cebu for at least two months. I never heard just what it was that prompted him to travel so abruptly, and no one volunteered an answer. When he later returned, he and I became the most cooperative of co-workers and the water question never came up with him again.

It was never necessary to call on the ghost again. The laboratory remained haunted. While an occasional knowing smile and a glance in my direction would accompany any reference to the ghost, the subject seemed to lose its fearfulness to the staff. It remained this way through the years of my relationship with the laboratory.

One day, the time finally came for my final separation from Cebu and the research program. I was in the U.S. at the time the decision was made by the directors of the Leonard Wood Memorial. A cable was sent to the island informing the staff of my "retirement." It went on to say that I would be arriving soon, in June 1983, for one last visit and to terminate my affairs.

I will never forget that last long slow trip up the road to the circle of administration buildings and to the laboratory.

In the building everyone was in tears. I had great difficulty avoiding tears of my own.

After several hours, I had completed the final details of my visit and had experienced too many tearful good-byes. I was cautiously approached by a group of my staff members with the query, "Did you not notice anything as we drove here on the road?"

"No, why?"

"Look out your office window, sir."

"Yes?"

"Look at your tree sir."

Now excitedly, "Good Lord, where is it?"

"It is gone."

"Gone where?"

"The day that your cable about retirement arrived, the tree caught fire. We tried to save it, but the fire was in its heart, sir. We even called the fire company and they became angry because we asked them to put out a fire in a tree, sir."

"Why did you not cable me to let me know?"

"We were afraid that you would take it as an omen, sir."

I slowly walked out of the laboratory, and everyone's eyes followed me. By the time I reached the tree, I had a crowd. They formed the usual silent arc behind me.

The tree was lying down. It had fallen across the road and its upper branches had been removed to open the roadway. The casualness with which the people regarded the fallen giant left little doubt that the ghost was no longer there. Two men, each on an end of a huge two-handled saw were slicing the great trunk lengthwise into four-inch-thick sections from root to crown. They stopped sawing and stepped back into the crowd as I approached. The three nuns also came and silently joined the others. It seemed that the entire population of the leprosarium had been waiting for this moment.

I had the stage to myself. I stood silently for a long time. I slowly walked up to the tree, hesitated, then broke off a sliver of wood protruding from the trunk and just as slowly carried it to a young tree next in line along the road. Placing the sliver of wood in a notch of a branch, I said, loud enough for all to hear, "Now, you will be my tree." As I walked back to join the spectators, I could see from their expressions that what I had done was right.

The nuns were all trying to talk at once. Mother took charge. "We did not know how you would feel," she said. "A caretaker was burning leaves on the bare ground next to the tree as it has always been done. This time, for some reason, the roots caught fire. The fire followed the root and burned into and up the center of the tree. We did not know what was happening until the fire broke out in flames at the top of the tree. Then we could not save it. However, we want you to know that everything is well. It burned all day, and many people just stayed here to watch it burn. It finally fell. As it was falling everyone around the area heard the sighing of many, many children. Some say they even heard the sound of your name."

I had told my staff that I wanted no gifts on this final visit. They did not completely follow my orders. As I was leaving the laboratory for the last time, I was given a small gift wrapped package. I objected, but they insisted. The package contained a three inch cube of wood. This block remains on my desk where I see it every day. On one side is inscribed my name and the statement: "This block is from your TIPOLO tree." The block also carries the signatures of the entire staff. The top bears the words, "We love you."

Six

The Search for a Cure: Jose Ramos

If the patient Dalmacia had the attributes for sainthood, then the patient Jose Ramos was a prime candidate for whatever lies at the opposite end of the spectrum. The nuns were constantly clucking their tongues at his behavior. They described him, with the kind of tolerance typical for nuns, as being naughty. However, they used the term "naughty" with obvious affection.

Joe lied, cheated, stole and whatever. This behavior was understandable. At the time of his birth, about twenty-odd years before I met him, his parents were patients in the large leprosy colony on the island of Culion. Around he time that he was born, this was the largest colony of its kind in the world. Most children of leprosy patients never become clinically infected but are, nevertheless, socially affected throughout their lives. Joe was one of those few children who contacted the disease as well as the social stigma.

If a child develops the disease, the symptoms usually become evident at five or six years of age. This is young enough that they can and do develop the skills that will be necessary for them to survive in life. They survive in spite of the handicap of having a disease that for little logical reason, especially in children, frightens people. These children, because of this public fear, have few options at a career.

Joe became a master beggar, the major profession that history has assigned to these people. He used his leprosy as a public attraction and often as a threat to plead for the charity necessary for his survival. Believe it or not he was most likeable. He was missing his top two front teeth, and this contributed to an appearance as a mischievous six-year-old. In spite of the missing teeth, or perhaps because of them, he had a smile that brightened up any room he was in. He behaved with admirable manners. He used "please," "thank you" and "you're welcome" far more often than the average person, and like a puppy dog, he tended to be overly expressive of his appreciation for even the simplest of favors. He was an obvious extrovert.

Nearly everything about Joe was the opposite of Dalmacia, including his leprosy. It was most difficult to conceive how their individual maladies could be given the same name. I only new Dalmacia as a bed patient. I never knew of Ramos as being confined to bed, at least not a bed in the infirmary. The leprosy of Dalmacia left her weakened, crippled, bedridden, but smooth of skin. Ramos was as physically competent as any healthy person of his age; however, the appearance of his leprosy fit the textbook description in every detail. His facial features were the epitome of the so-called "leonine" and he had no smooth skin anywhere on his body.

It was this classic appearance that brought him to my attention. He was selected as the subject for one of our routine weekly staff seminars. The descriptive comment when he was introduced to the professional staff included the remark that this was the way leprosy looked in the old days. Joe had been stripped of his clothing except for his jockey shorts and a T-shirt which he was allowed to keep in deference to the chill of the late afternoon. He paraded in front of the medical unit of the hospital like some candidate for a Ripley's museum display. It was obvious that he was actually enjoying every moment of the experience. The broad grin remained on constant display, and his behavior left little doubt that he had made appearances at medical seminars before. He demonstrated his long experience with medical examinations by anticipating our requests, frequently exposing areas of his body before we asked him about them.

I was interested in his tongue, mouth and throat. The wounds that he had in these places were of a kind that I had never seen before. I think that I asked him to open his mouth, stick out his tongue and pull up his T-shirt at least three times during the seminar. He was happy to comply, and it was clear that he became aware of my interest in these problem areas. Every time that I turned toward him, he immediately opened his mouth, stuck out his tongue and pulled up his T-shirt. I didn't mind too much. In fact it became funny, but this act became a habit that continued throughout the twenty years that I knew Joe. It became a sort of greeting. When he saw me approaching, even on the street, Joe opened his mouth, stuck out his tongue and pulled up his T-shirt. He used this means to keep me informed of his medical progress. In later years I gave thanks to Divine Providence that my early interests did not include his exposed buttocks.

Over the weekend following the seminar, Joe haunted my mind. His pleasant, happy character was not consistent with the great extent and duration of his disease. Any person with Joe's problem could have been forgiven for feeling sorry for himself. It was very clear that Joe was not sorry for himself.

First thing on the following Monday morning I sent a messenger into the hospital area to have Joe sent to me. Less than an hour later, the answer returned that Joe was not available. He had not been admitted to the institution. I was appalled and immediately set about to get an explanation. In response to my question, "Why did you not admit him?", I got a simple answer in the form of another question, "Why admit him, sir?"

Joe was considered to be an example of the development of drug resistance in leprosy. I was told that his leprosy had not responded to many years of the standard treatment. The explanation for not admitting him was as simple as the response that answered my previous question: "There is nothing that we can do for him—he will die within the coming year anyway."

One of the many difficulties to which one must become adjusted in the process of living in a less complicated society is the stark, basic, but nonetheless true and practical treatment of reality. The Ramos problem was a prime example of a simple truth of the kind that I could not bring myself to accept. I wanted to scream that this is turning your back on a problem; however, in this instance, authority had spoken. There was very little possibility that direct opposition to this decision would do anything more than solidify its certainty.

I had been trying for several years to get an experimental trial of a new drug at Eversley. A colleague, whom I admired much, had spoken to me at length about the possibly beneficial effects of a new compound. The drug was a modified dye, still refered to by its number B663 in a series of drugs, synthesized by an Irish chemist for investigation to be used against tuberculosis. His own laboratory tests in animals had shown that this new compound was safe and could be effective in leprosy in humans.

In response to my many requests, my Filipino colleagues, without exception, were adamant in their opposition to such a trial. The only argument that they had against the trial was the observation that the drug was a dye and it stained the patient's skin red. The red stain was not permanent; the color disappeared in about three months after treatment was completed. However, permanent or not, the property was considered most undesirable. I was told, "Even if the drug is effective, the patients will not take a drug that stains their skin red, so why bother testing it?"

The constant refusal of my request for a limited trial of B663 become a burr under the saddle of my existence in Eversley. I now had two burrs, the drug test and what to do about Joe. I decided to try to put them together. With my fingers crossed, I asked, "If Joe is going to die anyway, is there any objection to putting him on a trial of the red drug?"

I could tell that I had scored, not changed my associates' minds, but I had finessed them with their own argument. I got a not-too-enthusiastic approval, but as usual with a condition. Before we could try the new drug on him, Joe would go through a trial period using the standard drug, DDS. That would confirm his resistant leprosy. Since everyone knew that he would not respond to DDS, it was ethical that we must combine it with streptomycin, an antibiotic of potential effectiveness. Everybody agreed that this preliminary trial with the two drugs should take one year. If Joe did not improve in that time, then I could try the red drug. However, all parties concerned felt that such a trial would not be possible because streptomycin "is too costly and we don't have the money to obtain it."

The streptomycin requirement was an obvious ploy to bypass my request since its antileprosy effect had already been reported as being doubtful. In addition, certain of its side effects did not permit its use for extended periods of time, certainly not for a period of one year.

Not be outdone, I suggested that I would be willing to supply the antibiotic using funds from the laboratory budget. After a considerable, almost embarrassing pause, it was decided that we would test the new drug if I provided the antibiotic, and if I could get enough of the new drug for adequate testing.

I did want to test the new drug, but a preliminary trial of one year of regular treatment seemed rather long to me. Earlier, these same people had told me that Joe had less than a year to live. I decided not to make an issue of this timing for the moment. I had been outmaneuvered for a trial of the red drug, but I did succeed in having Joe admitted, on a temporary basis, to the hospital. You win some and you lose some.

Joe Ramos entered the institution and was embarked on a one-year preliminary evaluation prior to a limited investigation of the new drug. All of this was described to Joe in English, which he spoke well, and in the native dialect, which he spoke but rarely used. As might be anticipated from the general lack of desire to test B663, Joe's indoctrination into the program nearly always used the negative approach: "You don't really want to do this, do you?" Joe was not swayed. Joe knew a good thing. His usual response was, "I will be pleased to be the one who makes the sacrifice for those who follow." Joe was neither pioneer, humanitarian nor hero. He was a master survivor. Joe sure knew how to turn a phrase.

The one-year pretrial procedure began without further incident. It is safe to assume that no other patient in Eversley was receiving the attention that Joe received in his role as the sole member of a new drug trial. Rumor had it there were several Joe Ramos betting pools in the institution. The hard money was betting that Joe wouldn't make it. Within the first six months of the pretrial, Joe's condition began to worsen dramatically, and the betting odds against

Joe increased with time. There was no question that he was not improving and his condition required increasing amounts of medical attention.

Joe's health may not have been improving, but that did not seem to slow him down. He was in constant trouble with the law and with the hospital administration. He wandered from one misdeed to another.

One evening in the city, he was caught stalking around inside of the monastery of an order of priests. Nothing was done except to eject him from the premises. Next day it was discovered that the nonclerical clothing of one of the young priests was missing. In their place was an assortment of rather ragtag garments. Joe was later apprehended in the city walking around in the missing street clothes of Father Valencia. The good Father did not press charges. To remove further temptation from Joe, the priest arranged to provide Joe with more clothing. Henceforth, our experimental patient was considered to be one of the best dressed patients on the island. In deference to the hallowed source of his clothing, he was often referred to as Father Ramos.

The Ramos behavior became one of the most difficult parts of the scientific experiment in which he was involved. Too often, he did not show up for his routine examination and treatment because he was in the Cebu city jail for one misdeed or another. His presence in the jail caused the local authorities more grief than it did Joe. The other prisoners objected to his presence. Since I was the reason for his association with the hospital, it was my responsibility to solve Joe's problems. Either I or a member of my staff had to report to the jail and sign his release. No bail was required; the authorities were most understanding but they needed a signature to remove from them any responsibility for the act of releasing Joe into an innocent society. Joe never seemed to mind; he just grinned all the way back to the hospital and kept repeating how sorry he was and how he would now be good for ever more.

No one really took his promises seriously. His behavior was no better inside of the hospital area than it was on the outside. Joe found a lady friend and moved in with her and her husband. Both the lady and her husband were patients and had one of the small "nipa hut" family homes within the hospital compound. The husband was not well at all, so Joe took on with his status as house guest a great deal of responsibility. Among other things, he managed to help in the garden and do general repairs around the home. The husband and Joe really became friends. Not too long after Joe moved in, the husband died from his chronic illness.

Joe courted, won and soon married the widow. He later fathered a daughter who became the prime accomplishment, pride and most likely the sole property of any real value belonging to Jose Ramos. There was some question around the leprosarium about the timing of this birth. Some patients insisted that it was the child of the first husband; others said that it was an early birth. The wags in the institution looked at Joe and winked. When the child was baptized all eyes were on Sister Benigna who served as godmother. She later told me, "I knew what they had in mind. I just stared at Father McMahon during the entire ceremony and when he was finished, I handed the baby to Jose and told him to be a good father. Hah! they got nothing out of me."

During this period in the domestication of Jose Ramos, he pursued his profession of begging with a vengeance. He was now also responsible for a family. He did not remain true to his promise to be a good boy and I was still engaged in my perpetual task of keeping Ramos free from his frequent entanglements with the law. A few of his exploits were beyond immediate solution. One of these involved the nuns. When a blanket disappeared from a clothesline behind their residence, Joe as usual was the prime suspect. He protested loudly and clearly against the accusation and he was filled with self pity. "Every time something disappears," he said, "I am always blamed." This argument, however true, melted the hearts of the Sisters, and the blanket was written off as a normal part of their way of life.

The incident was forgotten, but not ended. A few weeks after it disappeared, the blanket was spotted by one of the Sisters on her way between the residence and the infirmary. It was hanging out to dry on the clothesline behind the home of one of the institution's nurses. The Sister immediately called Mother Superior who went to see the nurse and asked for an explanation. The explanation was simple. She had bought the blanket from Jose Ramos.

The blanket was returned to the Sisters by the nurse without further comment, but Joe was in deep trouble. He had spent the money and could not return it to the nurse. Jose Ramos was again incarcerated, but this time he went to the institution jail. The jail was nothing more than the hospital garage fitted with an iron grille that served as a door to the outside.

During this portion of the experiment in which he was participating, Joe received his food, medicine and medical examinations through the iron bars of his makeshift prison. The confinement was very successful. Joe was really being punished this time. He was not at all happy in this environment because his prison was more like a cage. His pride suffered. Everyone who passed could see him and laugh at his misfortune. It was the most effective punishment to which Joe was ever exposed. It was also a considerable amount of trouble to the institution and to the patient employees who had to care for him. About three or four weeks of catering to his whims were enough for all concerned. It was decided to free Ramos again on the promise that he would never again be a problem. I gave him a job as gardener and handyman to the laboratory. This gave him a modest income and, more to the point, kept him available for closer scrutiny.

After nine months of the preliminary trial, the patient really did become "a good boy." He was no longer very active physically and rarely smiled; his condition had become critical. I visited with him daily, but I had nothing to do with his clinical program.

One day I was so disturbed about Joe's condition that I asked to see his chart. When I reviewed it, I noticed that he had been given no streptomycin during the past month. When I questioned this omission, I was told that he had no more of the drug. I knew that was not true. I had provided more than enough of the antibiotic to last through the entire program. I am sure that I raised my voice in disbelief. I raised it high enough to assure everyone that I wanted some kind of explanation from someone. The excuses were many, and they came so fast that none of them made any sense. In the final analysis the primary reason for the missing drug was the fact that, "the drug was so costly and Joe was going to die soon anyway, so why waste such valuable medicine on such a useless case."

As heartless as that explanation may be, it was another example of a simplistic observation of a harsh truth. I called a staff meeting with a great deal more anger than my status allowed me to assume. If I got away with the outburst, it was testimony that my distress was very apparent and my colleagues were sympathetic to my grief. I requested a total examination and an immediate report on Joe's condition. I also asked that the preliminary trial should be discontinued and that treatment with the experimental drug commence as soon as the usual safeguards could be put in place. Every request that I made received prompt, unanimous approval.

If ever a drug test was initiated under adverse conditions, this trial of the red drug B663 certainly was. It would have been difficult enough to have tested Joe in the rather poor condition he was in when he first arrived, but now it looked hopeless. For Joe, what alternative was there? Rumor had it that the current betting odds within the institution were most unfavorable to Joe's future.

It was a fact; few patients anywhere were given the daily attention that Joe now received from the medical community. The trial that no one wanted had now become a challenge that everyone accepted. In response to the new drug, the color of Joe's skin gradually began to change from the beautiful natural tan of the Filipino to a deep red, almost black color concentrated mainly in the infected areas of his skin. With Joe, these were scattered over his entire

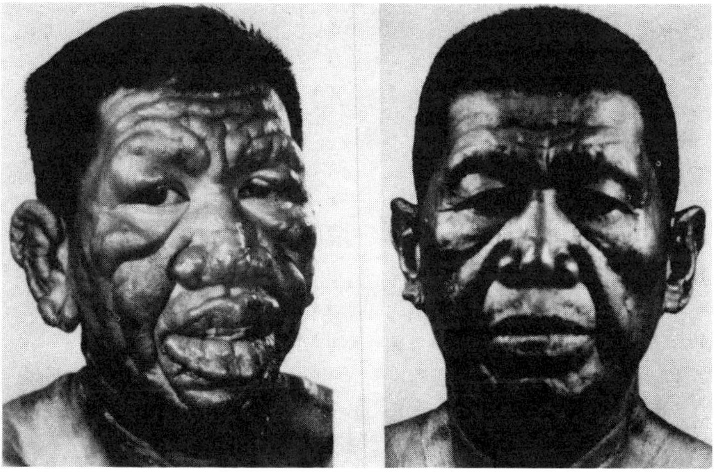

Ramos became black, but the color was of little significance; the fact was that Ramos began to improve markedly.

body. He turned black and around the hospital, the medicine soon was called "the black medicine." No matter what it was called, Joe changed color, but no longer seemed to be worsening. In fact, it became increasingly clear that he was improving. Within about three months Joe began to resume all of those bad habits and idiosyncrasies that had not exactly endeared him to the community in his earlier, active state of health.

Ramos became naughty again as his health improved and his skin turned black. Well, not actually black, but he slowly developed into the rich deep color of a dark cherry. The color was not uniform. It was concentrated in the places where his skin had seemed to be most in conflict with his disease. The areas between these sections were significantly lighter in color. The color between the dark areas was the kind of a tan that westerners pay good money to acquire in salons and on the beaches of the world. The color was of little significance; the fact was that Ramos began to improve markedly. Within six months the bettors were paying off the few gamblers who bet on Joe only because they couldn't resist the odds.

Six months after Joe started taking the experimental drug, a delegation of patients, including the mayor and members of the council from the patient government of the institution, came to see me. They gave me a petition requesting that other patients should also be allowed to try the black medicine. I called a meeting of the professional staff and presented them with the petition. I finally had the cards that I needed to promote a full scientific trial of the new drug. Everyone agreed and a new, scientifically designed experimental trial of B663 was approved. The trial would require at least eight new patient volunteers. There were more patient volunteers than we could accommodate with the amount of experimental B663 that was available.

Joe's improvement continued, and the darkened areas healed. The dark red color faded and fused into the lovely suntan color of the interim skin. Joe became noticeably lighter in color. He was admitted to Eversley as a permanent patient and was kept on B663 as his only treatment to check for the development of any drug resistance. He continued to improve and his color returned to more normal tones as he improved. In later years it was decided that the daily dose of the drug could be markedly reduced. Joe's infection showed no evidence of drug resistance in more than fifteen years of treatment with the black medicine. This fact is remarkable when one considers the very heavy bacterial

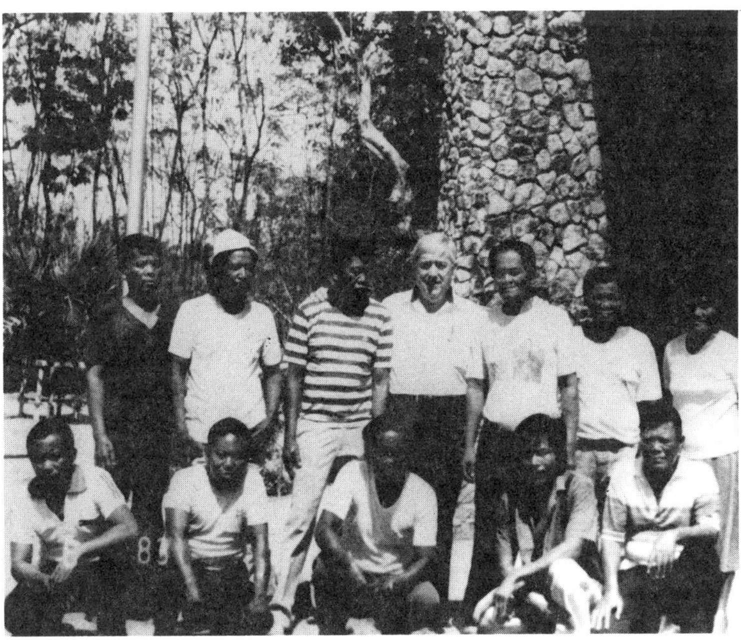

This group photo of the first B663 Experimental patients, taken on the last day of my last visit to Cebu, represents a major accomplishment in my life.

load that he was carrying when he first started on the drug.

Contrary to initial assumptions, the color was never a problem with any of the patients who took this medication. On my last trip to the Philippines, I had my picture taken with Joe and the group of eight patients who had been in the original experimental group plus a few others who had since benefited from its use. The eight original patients had been initially confirmed as having been failing on DDS, the standard drug of the time. As a result of their participation in the trial of the new drug, they were all well and showed little sign of their earlier disease.

The experimental drug has now been tested and approved in many areas of the world. It has been given the name "Clofazimine," a more respectable name than "the black medicine." Clofazimine is now one of the major drugs in the normal treatment of leprosy, especially the resistant type, throughout the world. This group photo represents a major accomplishment in my scientific career. I had disproven the statement, "Man would sooner be dead than red."

Seven

Leprosy Is a World unto Itself: Three Nuns

Dr. Jovellanos was the director at Eversley when I first arrived. This truly gentle person was the epitome of the gracious Filipino. He was indeed a gentleman and was approaching the age of retirement from the government service to which he had dedicated his lifetime. He administered to the needs of Eversley with an authority that was more evident in its effect than it was in its visibility. He issued orders with an obvious caution that gave evidence to his underlying fear of the patients' concern about the necessity for regulations.

Leprosarium directors, in general, were openly afraid of the consequences of issuing directives that might be unpopular with the patients. It is not easy to administer a population that includes the families of five hundred or more patients having a disease that does not sap their stamina. Patients in leprosy hospitals are confined but mostly ambulatory people—people who had to be antisocial to survive. Leprosaria are communities with their own unique set of social problems. To cope with these, the administrators establish their own personal police forces, usually one or two special patients with whom they can relate. These police are generally afflicted with all of the political shortcomings of their counterparts outside of the leprosarium. On occasion they have been known to shift their loyalties rapidly, especially when it was obvious that the majority of patients did not agree with them.

Once Dr. Jovellanos told me about an incident in the leprosarium at Jolo when the director gave an order that infuriated the patients. They, with the help of the unfortunate director's police, tied the director to a tree. During the night the patients built a campfire in front of his tree, and well within the range of his hearing, they sat around the fire, laughing and drinking a native beverage called "tuba." Tuba is sap from the coconut palm flower that is collected in bamboo containers placed high in the tree under the cut blossom. It ferments in the tree during the long, slow collection period. The alcohol level of tuba is usually rather low, but the drink becomes quite effective during an interval of drinking and conversation.

On that evening during the festivities, the patients discussed a number of possibilities for the director's future, which everyone loudly agreed would not be a long one. In the morning he was released unharmed and immediately resigned and left the area.

While some directors were wary of the power of the patients, there were others who, exercising the power of their office, established mini-dictatorships. This process is not difficult to conceive when you realize the extent of the political isolation of the leprosarium from the government of the people outside of its borders. As late as 1962, the director of a Philippine leprosarium had almost absolute power over the patient population. At that time, leprosy patients in the Philippines were wards of the state. They had no civil liberties, no vote, no access to the courts. This status has since changed; however, even today the irrational fear of this disease by the average citizen can produce social and legal isolation of the patients from the mainstream of the civil government. This, in turn, often produces quite unfair situations for the leprosy populations.

A good example of this misuse of power occurred in another institution not far from Jolo. The leprosarium at Zamboanga was located in an area that was a remote beachfront location, away from all other communities. As time went on, the population of the adjacent towns increased, and as they expanded their borders moved closer and closer to the leprosarium. Roads and transportation improved. Zamboanga, the "City of Flowers," became an international tourist mecca and the marvelous beach in the leprosarium outside of the city attracted increasing attention. The leprosarium location became more and more favorable. Soon it was more desirable as real estate than it was as shelter for the less fortunate, politically naîve patients.

One director finally moved the patients back into the hills away from the beach. He then built a series of cabanas along the fine waterfront part of the leprosarium. Friends of the director and politicians from Manila were given invitations to come to Mindanao and enjoy free holidays on the beach. All of this social grace was apparently financed by the leprosarium budget. Without doubt, this extravagance at the patients' expense solidified the national political power of the director. His invitations were eagerly solicited and he became known as "The Playboy of the Southern World."

In the course of time, the political activity on the famous beach in a leprosarium attracted enough public attention to cause a reassignment of the director. However, it also attracted attention to the fine entertainment value of the leprosarium property. The patients were eventually moved by the government, to a less desirable location. The old hospital grounds in the hands of real estate developers eventually became a popular and very profitable beach resort.

The morale of chronic disease hospitals has an inherent tendency to reflect the hopelessness of the problem to which they are dedicated. They share the isolation that society imposes on the disease leprosy. Not so at Eversley Childs. That escape from fate can be attributed to a great extent to the presence of the laboratory and its position of worldwide significance. The laboratory attracted numerous visitors from outside of the institution including scientists from around the world. This international visibility led to the implementation of more enlightened policies on the part of the government. However, while the laboratory focused the eyes of the leprosy world on Eversley, the unofficial presence of a priest and three unbelievable, elderly women—three Belgian nuns, named Benigna, Miguella and Rictrude—gave evidence that the ordinary people outside of the leprosy world could and did care what was happening inside of the institution. The nuns were the primary reason for the high morale of Eversley. They provided hope.

When I first met them, they were serving the people of Eversley in the old, full medieval regalia of their order. I was always amazed at the continuous physical application that was required to accomplish their routine chores around the hospital. I was appalled that this effort should be made under the obvious handicap of bulky and restrictive costumes in a tropical climate of such extreme heat and humidity. I eventually learned that the church is aware, that the church does correct, but that the church does take its time—a long time. The centuries-old style of the habits worn by these three marvelous women was finally changed to a much more efficient and comfortable garment during my stay in the Philippines.

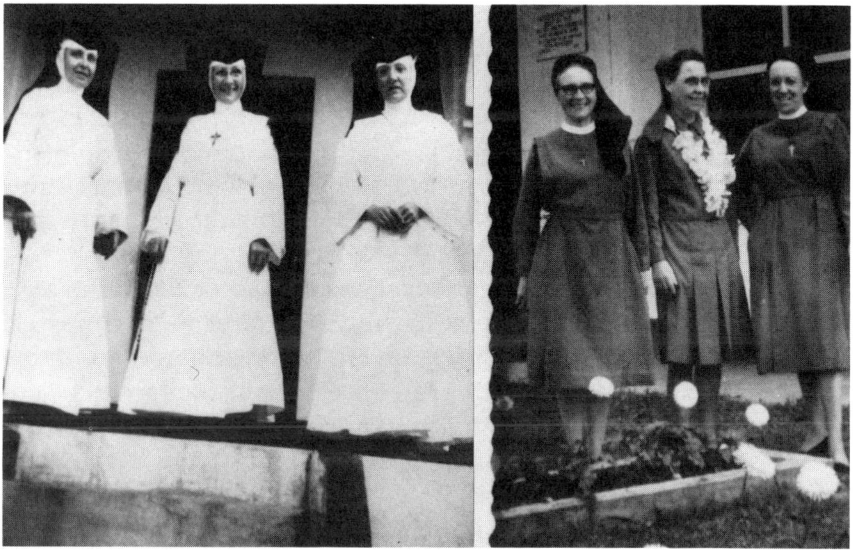

The centuries-old style of the habits worn by these three marvelous women was finally changed to a much more efficient and comfortable garment during my stay in the Philippines.
Old: Miguella, Rictrude, Benigna
New: Rictrude, Miguella, Benigna

I was not aware that I happened to be the only outside person available following the moment when the change of habit became official and acceptable. The moment occurred while I was in the laboratory after hours, sitting at the microscope table with no lights in the main laboratory behind me. I suddenly became aware of sounds, a tittering behind me, and I turned around to see three unfamiliar forms staring at me from the semidarkness of the outer room. The forms said nothing, just giggled. I finally said, "Yes, can I help you?"

This remark brought an outburst of laughter from the three figures. "You don't know us, do you, Doctor?"

The sounds were familiar, but not the figures. Finally, I thought that I recognized a voice and I haltingly asked, "Mother Rictrude?" Again another burst of laughter and they stepped into the lighted area saying, "We really fooled you, didn't we?"

Their gowns no longer swept the floor. They were attired in much simpler, yet still churchlike costumes that came just below the knees. Unlike the former bulky habits, the new garments allowed it to be vaguely evident that these dedicated persons were in the bodies of women. However, the most obvious change was around the face. The old costume had allowed only the very front of the face to be exposed. A tight white starched headpiece had previously pinched its way around their faces in front of the ears. Where this restrictive piece had been, their skin had never seen the bright tropical sun, but the exposed faces had become sun-browned and weathered. Now in the new costumes, wearing masks produced by the contrast of colors between the brown sunburned face and the newly exposed milky white skin of the ears and neck, the three nuns were strangers to me. The three masked women behind me in the shadow of a darkened laboratory bore little similarity to the sisters that I knew. Good enough reason for me not to recognize them. The obvious pleasure that they expressed at their successful deception made me glad that I hadn't recognized them.

It would be impossible to rank these women in some kind of a pecking order. They were inseparable and equally essential and helpful to the patient population. Miguella ministered to the needs of the male infirmary. These needs included acting as nurse, overseeing food preparation and distribution of medications, handling laundry, general cleanliness and sanitation—as well as attending to the spiritual well-being of her charges. Benigna did the same in the female infirmary. While she had fewer charges than Miguella, she had the additional task of delivering babies. Rictrude was the oldest. She was the contact with the outside world. She made sure that the materials were available for the proper conduct of the duties of the other two. She made the final decisions, but apparently never without approval of the other two.

Rictrude had been in service in the Philippines since 1926. She was Mother Superior by action and total agreement of everyone in or outside of Eversley Childs Sanitarium. I first came to be aware of the Reverend Mother in the period during the laboratory construction. I really got to know her while we were preparing for the ceremony for the inauguration of the laboratory.

The inauguration was scheduled for Valentine's Day, February 14, 1964. A ceremony with an international flavor was being prepared. There was a significant number of visitors with an interest in leprosy from many places around the world; scientists, physicians, administrators and others. It was an auspicious time for the program and especially for those of us who were directly involved in it.

The weather was typical for February in the Philippines, not too hot with a tendency to cloudiness and occasional rain ranging from misting to torrential in intensity. The misting rain played an important role in my introduction to Mother Rictrude and my future relationship with her.

The dignitaries began arriving for the dedication in the week prior to the big day. I was continuously escorting the visitors around the laboratory and the sanitarium. The new facilities were marvelous, and I was quite proud to serve as the new director and guide to these distinguished persons. On the third day before the dedication, it was raining enough to wet everything down, but not raining enough to stop the usual show-and-tell tour between the buildings. I was conducting a group that included my medical director, the president of the foundation and several visiting physicians from England when I took a very bad fall on the wet terrazzo tile steps leading into the clinic building. When I fell, the middle of my back hit a corner of the stairs and I slid breathless to the ground at the base of the stairs.

I certainly didn't lack for medical attention. Physicians were all around me. In a few moments my breath returned and on wiggling all of my digits, it was decided that the only casualty was my dignity. I continued on with the tour, apparently no worse for wear.

Except for a bit of stiffness, no other problem seems to have resulted from the fall; however the foundation president insisted that I was to go into the hospital as soon as possible to have X rays made of my back. He wanted to be assured that all was well. I agreed to do just that and we proceeded on toward the great event. The laboratory was to be properly anointed with no further reference to my mishap.

On the morning of the next day, following my embarrassing fall, I stopped at the local hospital on my way to the laboratory, and a good friend of mine, a registered radiologist who was also a diplomat of radiology, took the required X rays. I continued on to work with the promise that the friend would examine the photos and give me the results sometime during the coming day.

The rest of that day was a busy one. Most of the foreign dignitaries continued to shuffle around the facility, and we took advantage of their presence to review our future research plans with them. It was a challenging and rewarding day in spite of the intermittent and drenching tropical rainstorms that punctuated the day. It was raining like that as I closed the laboratory and headed for home, dinner and another cocktail affair that evening.

As I entered the garage next to the house, my wife came up to the car and asked if I had seen Nestor Canoy. He was the radiologist and no, I hadn't seen him.

She said, quite calmly, "Nestor wishes to see you as soon as possible. He was trying to get you all afternoon."

"I'll see him tonight—we are going to his house for cocktails."

"No, he says it is urgent and would like to see you before then. He stopped in here and he was quite excited. I think that you better run in to his office now."

"O.K., I'm off. Hold me a bit of dinner. I'll need something before I have a cocktail tonight."

I backed out of the garage and headed out of the compound in the pouring rain. I didn't get very far. About 100 yards from the house, I was just leaving the compound, when Nestor, driving from the opposite direction, met me at the gate. We both stopped our cars in the middle of the gateway, blocking it completely. Before I could respond, Nestor was out of his car and standing in the pouring tropical rain next to my car. I opened my car window and asked him to step into the car, but he immediately began to chatter at me with the rain wetting him completely, rain that was so heavy that it was soon dripping off the tip of his nose.

"Claude, you have a serious problem. I must discuss it with you."

"Come back to the house first and get out of this rain."

"No, this is fine, don't worry about the rain. This matter is too serious. Claude, those X rays showed that you have a massive abdominal tumor."

"Oh . . . oh!"

"I just want to ask you to stop in at the office for more studies as soon as possible, but most of all, I wanted to tell you about this before the cocktail party at my house tonight. I have already discussed this with your medical director, and I wanted you to hear it from me before you heard it from anyone else."

It set me back a bit and I finally said, "Is there any possibility that you are wrong."

"I'm sorry to say that it is not very likely that I am in error. I had taken a good number of views, and they all showed the same thing, a tumor about the size of my clenched fist. I also thought very seriously about this matter before I considered telling you. That is why I spoke to your medical director, Dr. Binford, first. It was his opinion that we needed to tell you as soon as possible."

Slowly, very slowly, I took a deep breath and said, "Thanks Nestor, I really must think about all of this first. I'll see you tonight. Perhaps I can have some plans by then."

Nestor, now soaking wet, patted me on the shoulder and slowly turned to his car, got in and, with a wave of the hand, turned around and drove away. I continued to sit in the car and stared through the rain for a few moments. Then somehow, I got the initiative to turn the car around, and I slowly drove back to the house. Val was waiting at the door. It was obvious that she had been told earlier.

That evening my tumor was the centerpiece of the cocktail party conversation. At least half of the men at the affair were physicians. Filipino, European and American, here to attend the coming laboratory dedication. Nestor had an office in his home, and after dinner he asked all of us into the office where he placed my X rays in the viewing frames for all to see and comment. The shadows and light spots that Nestor indicated as evidence of my problem really meant nothing to me, but I took little comfort in the fact that everyone seemed to be in agreement with his decision.

The medical director of the foundation, Dr. Chapman Binford, turned to me after the presentation and simply said, "What can we in the foundation do?"

I said that as far as I was concerned it was too early to make any final decision. First we had a laboratory to dedicate, and then we could discuss my problem. My immediate thought was that I would most likely want to return to the U.S. for medical attention.

Dr. Binford said, "Just let us know what you want and when you want it."

Next day at the laboratory, we were still in preparation for a dedication ceremony that was scheduled for the following day. However, news of Dr. Reich's tumor had spread throughout the land. Everyone greeted me with some form of assurance of their sympathy for my condition.

Sometime during the morning, Mother Rictrude asked to see me in my office. She was marvelous. She said, "Doctor, I have heard all about the tumor and I wanted to see how you were living with the knowledge of the difficulty."

I said, "Mother, while I certainly have a hollow feeling in my stomach, there is little that I can do about it. My immediate concern is to get this laboratory in operation; then we will see how badly I feel."

"Doctor, please do not let it cause you too much grief—the Lord will provide. I will give you my prayers."

I am not too sure how I felt about that. I am too much of a pragmatist to think too much about her words, except that her kind sympathy was most welcome and did make me feel better.

So, the next day we dedicated a laboratory and the following day was spent entertaining the many visitors from around the world. We were kept busy showing our guests the facilities and discussing the plans for the future research. Cocktail parties in the evenings took even more time, but no matter how hard I worked and how busy I was, there was always that very difficult time in the middle of the night when my mind would insist on dwelling on the medical problem that was confronting me. I can honestly say that no matter how unconcerned I tried to appear, those nights were among the most unforgettable moments in my life.

Finally, the guests were gone, the festivities were over and I was left with a newly dedicated laboratory to operate. That first morning, after the festivities were over, should have been the beginning of the challenge that brought me to this place, but before that there was a task to perform, a task that would determine the course of the rest of my life. I headed for the hospital and Nestor's office to have the X rays taken that I would take with me, back home to the United States. These would decide what I did next with my life.

Nestor was waiting and met me with considerable concern. He was a friend and he outdid himself in the amount of radiology that he accomplished. He was most determined to demonstrate every possible angle of the tumor that he was certain was present. The ordeal was not pleasant for me, and I couldn't wait to get away from the infernal machine that was making pictures of something that I didn't want to see. I finally left, with Nestor's assurance that he would contact me as soon as he had processed the film and read the results.

It was a very long morning at the laboratory. Before noon, the phone rang and it was passed to me. It was Nestor. He said, "Claude, I don't know what to say. I can find nothing at all in these pictures. There is no evidence whatsoever of anything resembling a tumor."

Much more was said than that, but the rest of the conversation doesn't matter. All that I heard was—there was no tumor. He couldn't explain it. Nestor said that he had rechecked, and he would still have made the same earlier diagnosis on the basis of the first X rays. I guess I could have been angry for the three days of anguish resulting from that diagnosis, but somehow I felt no anger, only a great deal of relief.

I walked out of the laboratory and could think of only one place to go. I headed to the house of the nuns. Mother Rictrude met me at the door and ushered me in to the small sitting room just inside of the porch. She had a tall glass of ice cubes ready and began pouring me a large, very large Scotch. She handed it to me then turned and said, "Yes, Doctor, now tell me what they found."

I said, "They found nothing, Mother."

She looked at me for some time and finally, almost in a whisper she remarked, "Thank God! You see, Doctor, the Lord really does provide."

It seems that Mother Rictrude had spent the three days of my ordeal in prayer and had the entire patient population involved in a prayer sesson on my behalf. The information that no tumor was found did not appear to surprise her at all. I don't believe that I ever will understand. There are all kinds of possible explanations and rationalizations for the experience that I had just had. For every explanation there is also some reason why that explanation is not quite satisfactory. As a scientist I don't know which one to select. I just know that, as I said before, Mother Rictrude was a remarkable woman.

Eight

Not to Sleep, Perchance a Memory: The Philippines

THE CARABAO

The Philippine version of the water buffalo is called a carabao. It is a massive elephant-gray ox with a pair of ebony black horns that can extend for more than six feet from tip to tip. In one of the pastures along the road to the laboratory, there is always a group of carabao being grazed while fastened to tethers. It amazes me that a carabao, with his strength and insensitivity to pain, would not merely pull up the tether that holds him. It is usually no more than a small stake that is just pushed into the ground by hand. That failing, why does he not just stroll off and break the slim rope that holds him to the stake? Occasionally one does wander off and if he decides to cross the road, he has an indisputable right of way. Any car that hits one of these animals is finished.

Among the group of carabaos in this particular field is a young, white carabao. He is actually pure, lovely white and is an impressive sight. I have often thought that if I ever were to write a book about the Philippines, I would entitle it *White Carabao*.

The carabao is solid, slow, persistent and very, very firm on the ground. He can be handled by a child. Often is the time I've seen a chain of the huge, gray, long-horned oxen, connected nose to nose by flimsy ropes, plodding along the side of the road; all of them under the control of one small girl riding on the back of the lead animal. The carabao can run, but he seems most uncomfortable when he does run. The motion is a kind of choppy, rolling gait, short-lived and awkward. When he isn't pulling the plow or hauling a cart, he is obviously quite contented with standing in the rain or wallowing in the filthiest of mud holes to escape the insects and the heat of the sun.

Under this mildest of manners, I am told lurks the wildest of emotions. The tales of the damage wrought by a mad carabao are hair-raising. However, there is no organization to the expression of his anger and for this reason, he is seldom seen as angry. His is usually a docile demeanor. The end result of his anger is nearly always his death when

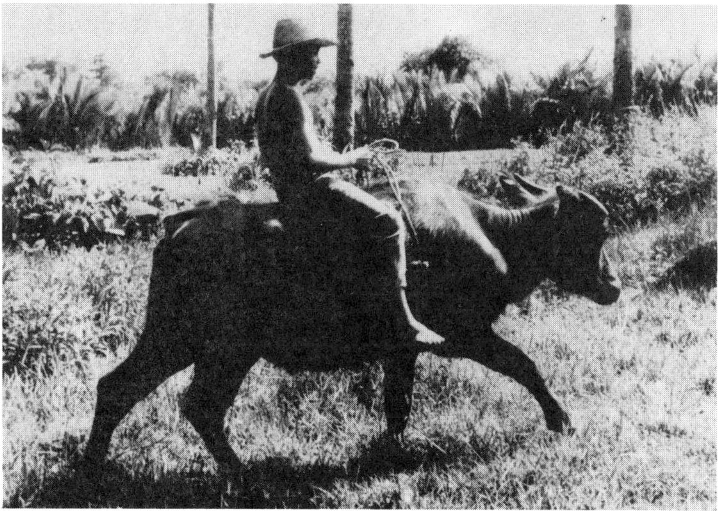

The Philippine version of the water buffalo is called a "carabao." The carabao is solid, slow, persistent and very, very firm on the ground.

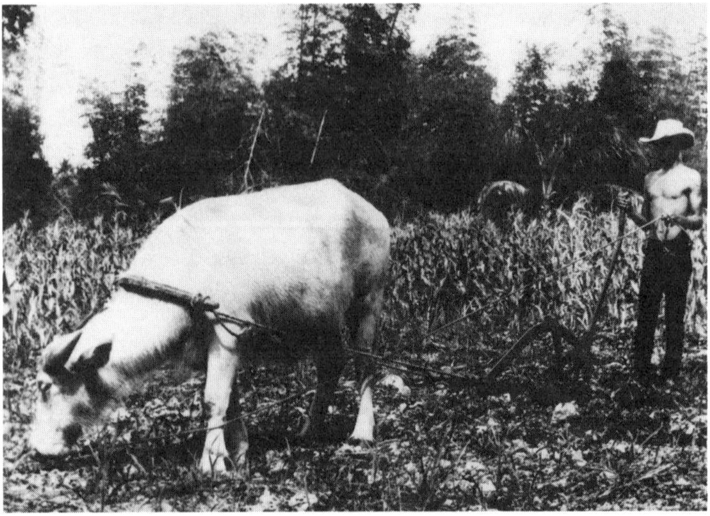

Among the group of carabaos in this particular field is one white carabao. I have often thought that if I ever were to write a book about the Philippines, I would entitle it *White Carabao*.

he runs into an uncompromising object and gives answer to the old query: "What happens when an irresistible force meets an immovable object?"

THE PEOPLE

If any animal can be representative of any nation or group of people, the carabao is amazingly a representative of the Philippines and its people. The Philippine people are marvelous. If I would be given the opportunity to select my nationality and race, I would almost certainly choose to be a Filipino. They have a beautiful story that they tell about themselves and about racial color preference. The story implies that the Lord himself would have made such a choice.

It seems that when God was making man, he first molded the figure and then put it into the oven to bake. On the first attempt the oven was not set high enough. The man was white and undone. So, God released his creation into the world and turned up the oven for another try, but the second time He set it too high and the man made in that effort was overdone and black. Knowing what He wanted, God reset the oven and this time it was just right. He had created the Filipino.

That beautiful suntan color is not the only reason for my partiality to the Filipino. I have never met more gracious people anywhere else in the world. If you are a friend, and friendship comes easy, there is no limit to the hospitality that they will shower on you. That hospitality often comes complete with lace tablecloth, crystal glassware, beautiful china, silver service and overwhelming attention to your comfort and appetite. Even the poorest of families have been known to put themselves into considerable debt in order to satisfy demands on their hospitality.

On the other hand, they also have a strange lack of sensitivity to living things that is hard to understand. There are no song birds here, not even any sea birds. Can you imagine an island where fishing is a major occupation, yet there are no gulls? Can you imagine an island of lush green vegetation and thick dark green, shiny leafed trees but no chatter of birds? The Filipinos' numbers and skill with the rifle and slingshot are a good part of the reason. They will kill anything that moves.

One fascinating pastime of young Filipinos is to catch a sparrow-like rice bird in a net and then tie a short string, about one to two feet long, to one of its legs. He will then tie the fluttering bird to a perchlike branch coming off the thinner end of a small limb, broken from a tree. The limb is usually about five feet long, perhaps an inch in diameter at the base, and it forks into two short branches each a foot long at the outer end. One of these branches becomes the perch for the captive rice bird.

This "bird-on-a-stick" is used as a walking pole. As the boy strides, pole in hand, the bird flutters up off the branch with every step. I imagine that to the youth, this creature has the fascination of the feathered papîer mâché whistling bird on a string and a stick commonly sold at carnivals in the West.

The fascination that I may have had with this act in the morning can disappear by the evening when the bird is completely exhausted, and he merely dangles on the end of the string gasping for air. I never heard of a bird being let go in exchange for the hours of entertainment that it provided to the child. However, this same child might often have been given the job of scaring these birds out of the fields to keep them from eating the family's rice crop. The rice bird is after all a pest that feeds on the main source of food of the people. This fact might justify the child's behavior.

In the center of many paddies there is a small shelter built on stilts, above and overlooking the field of rice. Long strands of thin rope span the distance between the shelter and the tops of tall poles planted along the borders of the rice field. To these ropes have been tied tin cans, metal strips and bells and any other available noise-making or attention-getting object. It is the task of the children to man these lookouts during the period when the rice is approaching the time for its harvest. As the rice birds flock down into the field to consume the maturing grain, the child pulls on the ropes to set the dangling objects in motion. The clamor has been known to alarm even passing motorists and usually causes the birds to fly off to the next field. This procedure saves much rice for the family. The boy is expected to spend the entire day at this tiresome routine, every day until the grain is harvested. For this reason, his concept of the tiny bird as a pest and his lack of sensitivity to the bird-on-a-stick may be understandable.

MOSQUITOES

While birds may be scarce, mosquitoes are not. They are omnipresent, and you do become immune or perhaps a better word would be "adjusted" to their constant fascination with human ankles and wrists as feeding stations. Very often at garden parties the mosquitoes will form small clouds around the heads of the guests, but social events proceed with no obvious concern with the bothersome little critters. Mosquitoes are a normal state of affairs, therefore, why allow them to disrupt one's life.

The mere presence of the mosquito is not annoying, one can accept that without being compromised, but the fact that they are constantly flying into your face is provoking. These garden parties are usually candlelight, semiformal affairs on a patio by a pool and extending onto a lawn. Guests hold their cocktail glasses in one hand and in the other, kerchiefs which they keep slowly waving in front of their faces to keep the air free for breathing and drinking. Frequently, one guest demonstrates his charity to a fellow guest by waving the offending insects from in front of the latter's face or brushing the critters from sleeves without bothering to halt the conversation.

Some effort is often made by the hostess to minimize the problem by placing lighted "Lucky Tigers" under the tables scattered around the lawn. Lucky Tiger is the brand name of a Chinese mosquito repellent. It is nothing more than scented punk wound in a coil about the size of the heating element on an electric kitchen range. The coil is held in horizontal position on a small tin spike, one end of which fits in a slot in the center. The outer end of the punk is lit and burns slowly, giving off a slight smoke with an odor intended to discourage mosquitoes. I think the effect is in the eye of the beholder and "Lucky Tiger" mosquito coil is just another example of the gracious hospitality of the Philippines.

Insect spray does not appear to help at all. Oh, that statement may not be completely true. I have often tried to clear mosquitoes from the bedroom at night before retiring and I have managed to kill quite a few. However, it usually requires a direct hit from the sprayer to achieve a heart-rending death scene as the bug slowly drags himself through the liquid that has surrounded him and which keeps him stuck to the surface. He finally gives up the struggle. I suspect that they are killed mostly by drowning in the kerosene base of the spray and not by the active ingredient in the insecticide. Under these conditions, it is much more effective, less expensive and less offensive to the nose to hit them with a flyswatter.

There is an interesting phenomenon that becomes evident when one attempts to kill Philippine mosquitoes in the bedroom with a flyswatter. They do not abide by the rules of American mosquitoes, at least not those of the mosquitoes of Eastern Pennsylvania with which I am familiar. In Pennsylvania, it was sport on a pleasant summer evening to swing at a mosquito, miss and then, *wham*, get him by following through with the swatter, as he invariably attempts to escape by flying upward and is silhouetted against the lighted ceiling or wall.

It would seem normal that a creature that flies would

attempt to escape by rising upward, away from an earth-bound enemy—not so the Philippine mosquito. These needle-nosed creatures, just as invariably, plummet to the floor in a wing-vibrating nosedive. You immediately lose sight of them in the dark shadows and against the dark background of the floor. You know that your next chance at killing him will only occur when he again returns to the attack in his own due time and at his convenience. You can be sure that he will return and that he will be returning to the attack, silently from behind and below. I have had enough painful experiences in this respect to make me place my bet on the bug anytime. This curious behavior trait apparently has been bred into the local mosquito population as an extremely effective survival mechanism.

TASTES AND ODORS

Taste preference is one of the most noticeable of the differences between Filipinos and people from the West. First among these is the preference for rice over bread and potatoes. Many of my Philippine friends have told me that, for them, bread and potatoes are not satisfactory replacements for rice. No matter how much bread they eat they remain hungry until they have had some rice and, contrary to western concept, what these people consider to be good rice is not fluffy rice. The average Philippine rice pot contains a heavy, mushy mass of grain, cooked in the morning and served cold "en lump," as needed, from the same pot all day long. The rice pot in character and texture of its ingredients can be compared with the boiler of oatmeal that, in the early days of America, sat on the back of the stove all day long.

These people do not really care for the heavy sweet-tasting food of the West. The most popular Philippine candies are only moderately sweet to the Western taste, and that fact seems strange when one realizes that cane sugar is one of the major products of this country. The Filipino taste runs more to the aromatic, somewhat soapy and sort of sulfurous background foods. There is a popular fruit, native to Mindanao, one of the larger islands to the south, called durian; it is frequently available from pushcart vendors who call out their wares as they pass along the streets outside of the houses. I stress "outside of the house;" any Filipino will, with apparent pride, laughingly agree with you that durian has a strong odor; one might even say, it stinks. Even the Philippine airlines, a role model for such behavior, will not tolerate durian on board, neither to be eaten there nor to be carried as hand luggage.

Those who eat this fruit, and there are many, profess great joy at the flavor, which they say is marvelously different from the odor. I do hope so! The odor is beyond polite description. There appears to be a fruity pineapple-like carrier to the basic odor, but the pineapple concept is only momentary. The basic odor quicky overwhelms anyone who sniffs without warning. I never could rationalize the psychological or physiological forces behind this taste preference. In the West, we say that it was a brave man who ate the first tomato. I can say without hesitation that it took a far braver man to eat the first durian.

Dr. Victor Heiser in his book, *An American Doctor's Odyssey* tells the story about two Americans on a Philippine train, riding in a car in which a fellow passenger, a Filipino, was eating durian. The Americans complained to the conductor about the odor and without hesitation, the offender was made to eat his durian outside of the car on the platform. When he finished his Philippine delicacy he returned to the car and immediately complained to the conductor about the Americans who were eating their cheese sandwiches. They, in turn, ate their lunch on the platform. Turnabout is fair play.

Then there is balut! Balut is a duck egg which has been incubated to a point close to hatching. At the right moment in the incubation period, before the feathers harden, this unhatched egg becomes a delicacy that is savored and eaten—as is. It is sold by street vendors in much the same manner as "Good Humor" ice cream back home. In late afternoon or early evening, it is quite common to hear vendors call, "Balut, baaalloooot!" Considering the nature of the item, they do a remarkably good business.

Taste and odor are inseparable, and I suspect that these differences in the kind of tastes that are preferred are in some way related to the difference in the odors of densely populated areas in the cities of the Orient when compared to similar areas in their European counterparts. In America and Europe these odors repulse me. In Asia, they are not repulsive—they are interesting, possibly because in the East, I am not familiar with the substances behind the odors. There is no way to describe an odor except by comparison, and the best I can do with the odor of Oriental cities is that the base to the odor is not unlike the smell of raw potatoes pan frying in lard. On this basic scent is superimposed a subtle overlay of the mingled scents of vinegar, sauerkraut and wet newspaper.

There are other scents of some significance in the Orient. The odor of urine is inseparable from human habitation anywhere, but this is especially true wherever there is a concentration of people and a shortage of fresh water to service the public sewage facilities. We tend to forget that in a country like the Philippines with a population of close to sixty million people, there will be a release of something approaching one billion gallons of urine per year. That condition can and does contribute to some kind of an odor problem anywhere in the world, a "sea of pee," so to speak.

The men here urinate everywhere—against a wall, a tree, a house, in the gutter, usually without concern about covering themselves; turned away from the crowd, yes, but covered, no. In the morning, en route to work it is very common to see little boys standing in the front door of the house, peeing to the side of the doorway, sometimes on the walk. In many public buildings with a restroom, the odor of urine is strong enough to be obvious in the corridor, sometimes even to the sidewalk. I have actually seen an office in an old public building in Cebu, that had big black letters painted on the wall behind a row of men's desks admonishing all, "Do Not Urinate Here."

It is a familiar and awesome sight to see a big bus stopped along the road and all of the men on the bus are standing around the bus, "washing" the tires. The wall surrounding the house across the street from one of the houses in which we lived was a favorite "watering hole," because it was also a regular bus stop. The normal male behavior at this spot became commonplace and not worth mentioning, but sometimes the odor was not pleasant. It is an odor that I associate with this country. Most Americans spell Philippines with two Ls and one P; Phillipines. That is a mistake I never make anymore. I know that there is only one L and two Ps. "Pee" is for Philippines.

TRANSPORTATION

The jeepney is a fascinating vehicle. It is an outgrowth of the large numbers of military jeeps that were left behind by the U.S. Army after World War II. To this day, these are described by the older Filipinos as "MacArthur jeeps."

The urgent problem of postwar public transportation was solved, in part, by some ingenious individuals who extended the body of the "MacArthur jeep" and put a fringed roof on four posts over this rear extension. The original design has a front seat and a truck type back with two long benches along each open side. Passengers enter by way of two steps up into the rear center and sit facing each other toward the midline of the vehicle. Canvass curtains roll down from the roof in bad weather. A normal load would be six people in the rear, at most eight, but I have seen anywhere from twelve to twenty people, complete with baskets of vegetables, chickens and even pigs crowded into one immutable mass. The roof can provide freight storage space, and ocasionally, perhaps even support for a passenger or two.

The jeepney is by far the most popular means of local transportation, and these gadgets greatly outnumber anything else on the road. They are beautifully painted in bright, gaudy multicolors and have fantastic names ornately lettered on the front and sides. The names are not always, but usually religious in connotation; "Holy Mother of God," 'Señor Saint Narcisco," "Mother Help Us," "San Sebastian," and so forth. One time I was run off the road by a jeepney named "Have Faith in God." The same jeepney, another driver, did the same thing to me at the same spot on the very next day. "Have Faith in God"; I do, I do.

WEATHER

Did you ever consider the possibility that constant fair weather can be a pain in the ass? That description may sound crude, but in all honesty, I can think of no better way

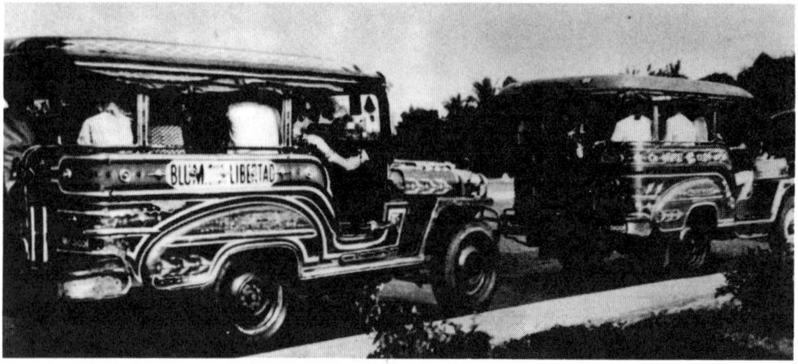

The jeepney is by far the most popular means of local transportation, and these gadgets greatly outnumber anything else on the road. They are beautifully painted in bright, gaudy multicolors and have fantastic names ornately lettered on the front and side.

to put it. Most mornings you see a blue sky flecked with white clouds and a white glaring sun. Evenings the sun goes down accompanied by a beautiful apricot sunset. As it is said in the song: "Sunrise, sunset . . . sunrise, sunset"; and on and on.

The most popular Philippine postcards show a carabao, a palm tree, a nipa hut and a Filipino native wearing the traditional broad brimmed woven grass hat of the farmer. All are silhouetted against an apricot sunset over a darkened glassy sea. It is true. There are a few exceptions, mostly during the rainy season, but somehow one gets the feeling that on every evening of the year there is a beautiful sunset, each one slightly different from the sunset of the night before. I heard the story told that an internationally famous newsman, when stationed in Manila, said that he had a friend who had spent a long time in the Philippines. One evening the friend reportedly looked up into the sky and said, "Oh no! Not another GD beautiful sunset," and shot himself. I myself have often thought longingly of a cold foggy drizzle that, happily, might last for at least umpteen days.

THE TYPHOON

The most noteworthy aspect of Philippine weather is the occasional typhoon. I think that typhoons look as bad as they do because of the palm trees. The trees sway, bending far over with the wind. The clusters of leaves topping each tree are blown full back exposing bunches of coconuts and the dry, brown middle of the leaf cluster. Standing together in rows and bending with the wind, palms in a typhoon look like rows of tall, slender American Indian chiefs in full headdress, bravely standing facing into the wind. Banana trees, the ordinary Indians, just get blown over, row on row.

During a typhoon, every modern facility on the island will be fully stressed by nature; unbelievably, most will survive. Many native nipa huts will be blown down and will roll down the roads like tumbleweeds over the prairie. The owners, with friends and family, will run after them in the rain. Usually, everyone is laughing and chattering as they secure the dwelling in some place where it will remain until they return, retrieve it, roll it back and re-erect it on its own stilts after the storm has run its course. Some foresighted natives, a few, will have propped their homes into the wind with long bamboo poles.

There is no serious attempt on the part of most of the people to keep dry. They just walk around, wading through the water up to their knees and often higher. In front of the small native stores, known as "sari sari stores," are huddled groups of men with the water pouring down their faces. They are obviously chatting about the storm and the effect it is having on the community. A young boy may be standing nearby in a stream of water in a gutter and, in the midst of a typhoon, he will be tossing fallen coconuts up the stream and retrieving them as they rapidly float back past him. Young girls, soaking wet, with their dresses clinging to their bodies, walk along the road, laughing, talking rapidly and using large banana leaves, held over their heads as umbrellas. It all seems like a giant picnic.

Trees fall across the road, but there is always some one or some group that clears the road immediately by cutting a path through the fallen giant. It is a moot point as to whether this task is done as an act of charity to one's fellow man or most likely to salvage the scarce firewood.

At places the torrent of water running from the hills to the sea will cross the road in a wide swift stream. With no other available way to detour, the motorist is faced with the decision to brave this way through the water to the clear road visible again only 50 or so feet away or sit it out until the water subsides. The water doesn't look that deep, but these roads are often not too well paved and the rush of water could have created a three-foot-deep pothole out there somewhere.

Groups of natives will gather at these places where the road disappears into the stream. The bystanders watch the drivers to see what they will do. They urge him on. When he inches into the current they applaud. If the driver decides to wait, he becomes an object of derision for his lack of daring. There is method to the madness of this roadside audience, because for a price, often a rather high price, especially if he does proceed on his own and gets stuck, the local natives will help the driver across the stream. He pays the price, shuts off his engine, releases his brakes and gears and the laughing, happy throng surrounds his car and half pushes, half lifts it through the water to the clear roadway ahead. The town mayor is usually agent and cashier for the crowd.

This profitable native business venture usually ends shortly after the typhoon. However, there has been at least one enterprising group in a village along the main highway who found a way to extend their good fortune. At one place along the highway, about halfway between the city and the favorite bathing beach north of the city, there was a spot where about one hundred yards of the road was always inundated during a heavy rain. The people in the village adjacent to this stretch of road built a dam up in the mountains above this point and collected the excess water during storms. During dry periods, the dam was opened and the water was slowly released, just enough to keep the highway flooded for several hours. The water release was usually well timed to prevent the "rich people" of the city from reaching their beachside cabanas on Friday afternoon,—except, of course, for the price of passage across the mysterious current.

It is noteworthy that this flood was not deep enough to stop the native jeeps or busses, just deep enough to cause hesitation to the drivers of Lincolns, Cadillacs, Mercedes and other luxury cars. The stream was, therefore, regulated to just the proper discriminatory depth. The price that was charged for the push was based on the urgency of the demand for the service and the apparent ability of the customer to pay for the service. Therefore, one could say that, based on character and pricing practice, this native car ferry was a prime example of venture capitalism.

The period after a typhoon is a letdown. All now finally becomes still, and the heavy, quiet, tropical air steams with humidity. In the hot, humid, calm air the mosquitoes swarm in thick clouds over every moving object, and people begin to become aware that the storm is now over and normal life must resume. They begin to put together the broken pieces.

The local radio station, because of downed power lines, will be heard only by those people with battery-powered radios which here are simply called transistors. Wherever someone has a good one, a cluster of people gathers around to find out how much damage was really done by the storm to the island. Sometimes the news is not good: A group of squatter homes on the southern edged of the city was washed away. Now there is concern for friends or families. Charity is necessary and people are rushing every which way to help where they can. In their eagerness, they get in

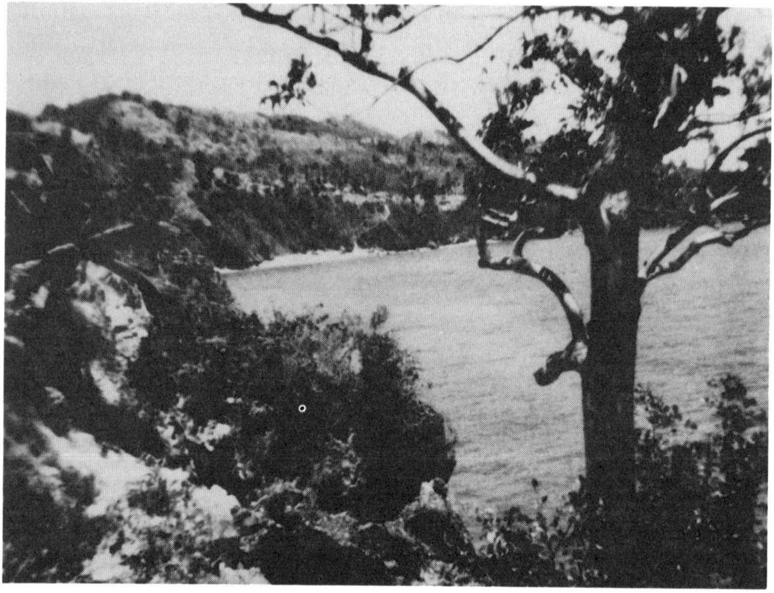

At some places, the road goes along cliffs high above the sea, and the view down the cliff to the narrow strip of beach and the tropical sea is like a fairy tale.

each other's way, hindering the effort. The local radio announcer says, "I am happy to announce that an *anonymous* donor, a certain Mr. A. C. Sixto, has just donated a box of clothings and the Cebu Bakery has generously contributed two cans of cookies."

Life eventually returns to normal. It will be some time, most likely days, until the power is restored to the island. The fallen wires are everywhee. People walk among the fallen wires as if they are nothing more than vines dangling from the trees. There is nothing to fear because the generators are not running, and it is certain that they will not be turned on again until the wires are picked up and the circuits are clear. To those of us more familiar with fallen, arcing wires and constant warnings to avoid fallen wires this behavior is maddening. Regardless of the lack of concern by the people around you, it is still quite a thrill to step over, on, or under fallen wires. As with the wires, the storm is soon forgotten.

SERENITY

If one drives far enough to the north of the city, along the main road around the island, one travels into the world of the Philippines of the past. An occasional native hut can be seen along the road, but the land and the available water supply will not support many people. While the land is harsh, it also becomes calmer and much, much more beautiful. At some places, the road, without guardrails, goes along cliffs high above the sea and the view down the cliff to a narrow strip of beach and a broad, sparkling, deep blue tropical sea is like a fairy tale. There is the faintest suggestion of other islands far out on the edge of the horizon.

Farther on, the plain between the mountain and the sea widens, and the road returns to sea level. The narrow beach borders on a shallow coral reef stretching out into the calm water. Up and down the coastline, one can see rows of sun-browned fisherman standing far out on the reef. They are out far enough that one must make a special effort to notice any movement. Otherwise, they are just rows of posts jutting out of the water. Still farther out, a few outrigger canoes with breeze-filled sails move quickly up and down the coastline. The hot, bright sun hurts the eyes, but here, unlike nearer to the city, the water is clear and the air smells clean and refreshing.

Nestled between the beach and the road, in a grove of palm trees, is a native village. A scant half dozen stilted, nipa palm-thatched huts circle a clearing in the center of which is a round and time-blackened firepit. An aged man squats by the coconut charcoal fire that is glowing under a browning pig on a bamboo spit. His only motion is a casual shift of the hand as he slowly turns the spit. This is his share of the daily chores in the community. All could be quiet and for best effect should be quiet, but the stillness is broken by the continuous din of happy noises from an unusually large number of small, brown, naked children running everywhere.

This is the Philippines that I love, unspoiled by a mad rush to accept Western culture. I have written of the difficulties of life in this culture. I know they find similar problems in ours. Filipinos can become terribly homesick in the midst of what we consider to be the glitter and glamour of the West. I understand their feeling. The West is my home, but I feel a sweet, longing ache when I think of the golden sunset, the carabao, the nipa hut, the fishing village and the Filipino people.

Nine

Alas and a Lei: Farewell

In 1982, twenty-three years after I first joined the foundation, a newer and younger administration with an eagerness to change direction ascended into its leadership. Shortly after the change of offices, the board of directors of the Leonard Wood Memorial announced my retirement. I was allowed to return to Cebu for a brief final visit to close out my affairs and to say good-bye. "Goodbye" is an English word that has few counterparts in other languages. The Germans say "*Auf Wiedersehen*," which is a synonym for the Filipino "*Ma balik ako* [I'll see you again]." Good-bye is forever. That makes departure so much more difficult than any other salutation. Everybody knew of the finality of my visit before I arrived, and the mood of nostalgia overshadowed everything during the entire several days of my stay. The visit bore some similarity to dying. I have not yet experienced dying, but I pray that the pain is no worse.

One of the longest trips I ever made in my life was the last trip from my laboratory in Cebu to the airport on Maktan, the small island adjacent to Cebu. Maktan is separated from Cebu by a narrow, navigable channel that has been crossed in succeeding generations by *banca* (the native outrigger boat), barge and bridge. This tiny island is little more than a coral and marsh flat that sits like a shield in front of Cebu City harbor. It has a considerable role in history as

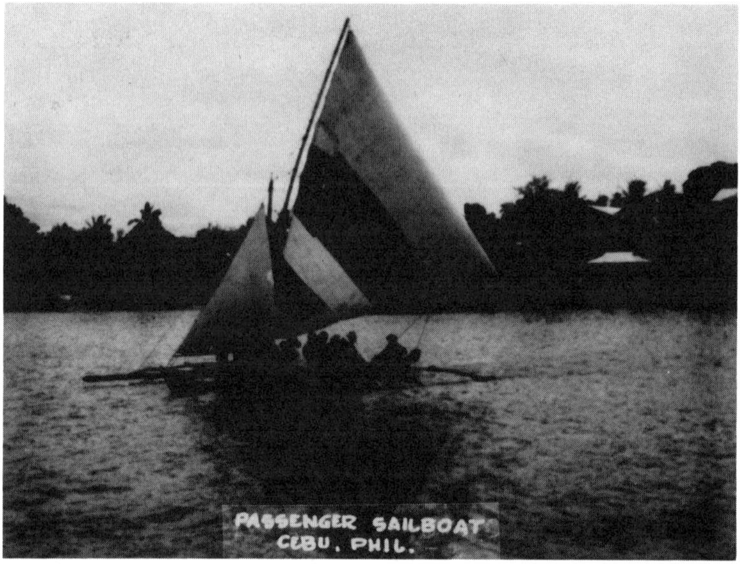

Maktan is separated from Cebu by a narrow, navigable channel that has been crossed in succeeding generations by *banca* (the native outrigger canoe), barge and bridge.

being the place where Ferdinand Magellan was killed, half-way around in the first-ever circumnavigation of the globe. There is an impressive monument on Maktan that marks the site of this event. The native chief who is said to have done the deed was named Lapu Lapu and today, in his honor, the largest city on the island has been given his name. In earlier, Spanish times, Lapu Lapu City was called "Opon." A marvelous airstrip was built on Maktan by the U.S. military just after World War II, and this was my destination, the airstrip that serves Cebu as a domestic airport.

Domestic airports are nearly always crowded. I say domestic as opposed to the international, several of which exist in this country; Manila International, Maktan and a few others bear this designation, but except for Manila, local international airports are mostly nonfunctional as such. This is not to say that international airports are not crowded—heaven forbid! In the Filipino language, the word "airport" must mean "crowded."

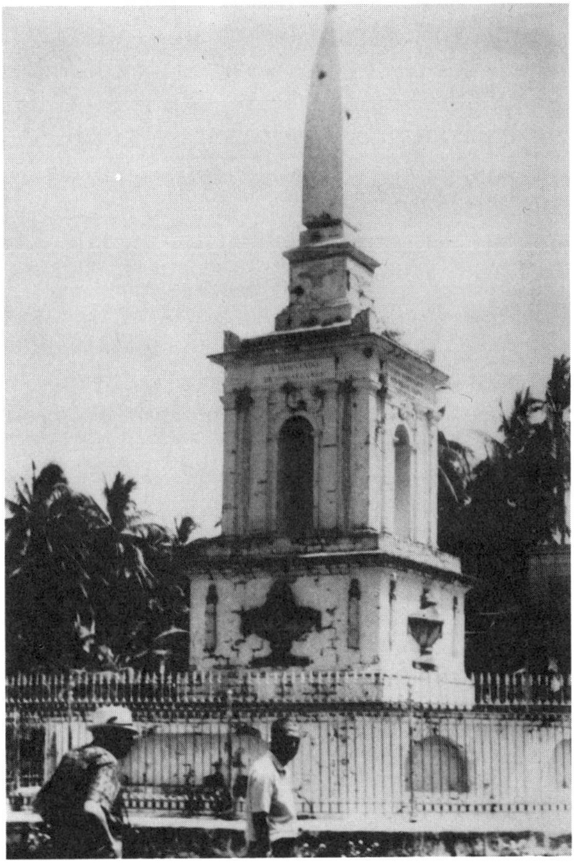

The Magellan Monument—Maktan has a considerable role in history as being the place where Ferdinand Magellan was killed, halfway around in the first-ever circumnavigation of the globe. There is an impressive monument on Maktan that marks the site of this event.

Domestic airport crowds, however, are different. They are more homespun, sparkling, more clean of face and far less formal—far less sophisticated than their international counterparts. Domestic crowds tend to concentrate into a much closer mass than the international variety. The domestic airport is more of a neighborhood function and as such, the departure is more like that of a guest leaving one's home. The departure lounge serves as the equivalent of the front porch of the house for leave-taking. Every individual in the crowd is doing their best to get as close to the departing guest as possible. The almost person-to-person contact is the last manifestation of love.

There are also other members of the crowd who are not seeing loved ones depart but are awaiting new arrivals. Their purpose in the crowd is not to say good-bye, but rather theirs is a mission of eager anticipation, of seeing a loved one again. They usually tend to form into happier, more social groups around the edges of the serious, frequently tear-eyed well-wishers.

They who are waiting congregate at the windows facing the airstrips or at the doorways through which arrivals will enter. Since the planes are nearly always late, the morning arrivals and afternoon departures quite frequently overlap, so that the people who are saying good-bye and those who are waiting on new arrivals intermingle. Very often, one who is waiting an arrival is made aware of a friend who is leaving, so he joins the well-wishers until his plane arrives. The entire airport ceremony is obviously a ritual carryover from the dockside greeting and leave-taking of the old days of sunlit sails slowly disappearing over the horizon.

Looking out over the airport throngs it is easy to spot the travelers. They are usually at the center of an inward-facing circle of friends, relatives and interested spectators.

All of those who are departing are bearing a multiple of leis of kalatuchi flowers, each lei placed around his or her neck by a member of the surrounding crowd. The thickness of the collar of blossoms is in direct proportion to the size of the circle of friends. Those travelers in the center of the

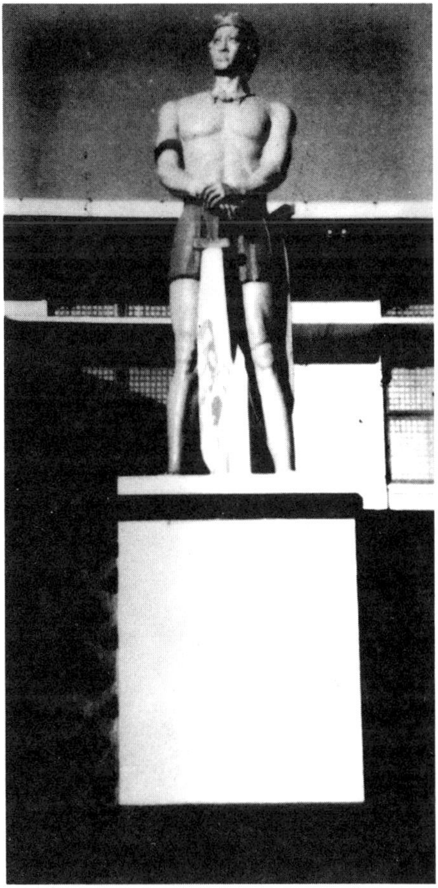

The native chief who is said to have killed Magellan was named Lapu Lapu, and the largest city on the island has been given his name.

larger circles bear mounds of flowers high enough to obscure their necks, chins and often their noses. This makes talking, even breathing a bit complicated. It makes good-bye kissing impossible. These are flowers with a scent heavy enough to fill tropical air. Heavy enough to cover the garlic, fish, fowl, sweat and assorted odors of the animate and inanimate cargo of the soon-departing aircraft.

The kalatuchi is also known as the cemetery bush because it is frequently found as a planted form of remembrance to the dead. The plant, sometimes called "bush," most often "tree," is usually about ten to fifteen feet high and equally wide with large paddlelike leaves that grow and fall with the seasons, which are otherwise obscured in the tropics. The flowers hang in thick aromatic clusters of finger-length, trumpet-shaped blossoms that can be plucked like grapes from the clusters. The leis are simply

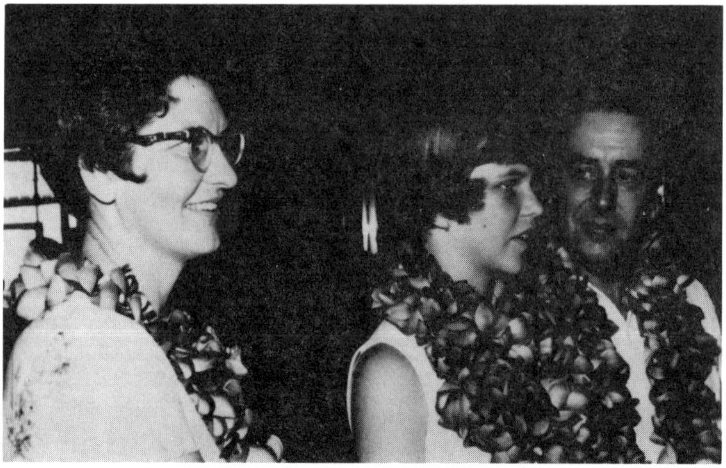

Kalatuchi blossoms—those travelers in the center of the larger circles bear mounds of flowers high enough to obscure their necks, chins and often their noses.

made by piercing the trumpets lengthwise with needle and thread. From the tiny end, through the blossom and out of the daisy-shaped bell, they are strung together like beads. Each tiny end is pulled into the center of the daisy-shaped bell of the previous blossom to form a chain of pink and white petals of delicate, cool and fleshy softness.

Eventually, the crowd begins to mill toward the boarding exits and the kissing and leave-taking becomes more animated as it becomes obvious that the soon-to-depart plane is boarding its passengers. Each well-wisher hangs on as long as possible, finally only maintaining touch with extended arms and fingers as the traveler passes, with difficulty, through the mass of people and out of the crowd. Those left behind resent the restriction that breaks their contact at the exit leading to the aircraft, but when contact is finally broken, an air of normalcy returns and each member of the crowd seeks a vantage point from which to view the takeoff. They won't leave until the plane is up and out of sight.

To the traveler, the long walk from the airport to the plane is a welcome respite from the dense mass of humanity in the lounge. The cheery welcome on board signals relief not only from the crowd, but also from the swelter of the tropics. The cool open doorway to the plane is a welcome sight, and the line of passengers, slowly mounting the stairs is usually slowed even more by the passenger who, finally reaching a desirable seat, is no longer concerned with the line coming up from behind. That line must now await his convenience as he slowly piles his carry-on cargo around him—on, under and over his selected seat. Fortunately, any competition for the unreserved seats takes place for the seats in the rear of the aircraft. Every local experienced flyer knows that these are the seats from which the survivors are taken in air crashes. This act certainly expedites front-end loading of the aircraft, in spite of the unbelievable amounts of personal luggage surrounding each passenger.

As one enters the aircraft, leaving the brilliant tropical sunlight behind, the interior coolness of the plane is made visible by the sequence of plumes of mist blowing from the cool air nozzles over each seat. The tropical humidity of the ground air is condensed by the cool air being forced from each vent. Sometimes the condensation is so great that the stewardess is required to walk up and down the aisles touching each vent with a wiping cloth before takeoff. This thoughtfulness prevents the passenger from sitting in a seat whose wetness would not have been evident to eyes just becoming adjusted to the dim light of the cool interior.

Finally, with everyone seated, the kalatuchi leis can be removed. It is unthinkable that one should take them off in view of the giver. Fortunately, departure is often delayed and this delay provides time for the odor of the kalatuchi to clear from the air in the plane and gives the traveler time to clear the odor from his nose. The delay is most welcome to the unfortunate flyer who is air sick prone, a problem that is made worse by the heady scent of the flowers.

The stewardess solves the problem of what to do with the leis by handing out plastic bags, and the masses of blossoms having achieved their purpose, are stowed away in the overhead rack. The blossoms will be wilting before the plane lands. Each lei, on removal from the bag, will seem to have too much thread stringing it together. It will not be placed around the neck again, but will not be left behind.

Ultimately the kalatuchi lei will be taken from its plastic bag. With thoughtful hesitation, the now-brown blossoms are finally disposed of in the hotel room wastebasket, but not without a soulful review of the life left behind in the domestic airport crowd. In the cool darkness of the first

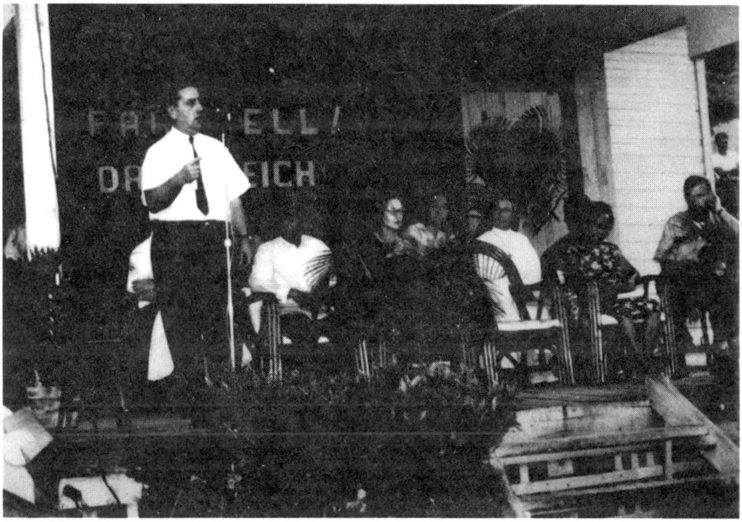

"Farewell, Dr. Reich!"

night away from the love of its donor, the kalatuchi lei becomes a rosary of memories, each blossom a prayer that those memories will be relived again, that the sparks of the love and the life left behind will always glow with the same intensity. It is a lovely prayer, but the flowers are put away with the sad certainty that the memories will slowly become faded like the blossoms from the kalatuchi.

Appendix

BIOGRAPHICAL
Claude V. Reich, Ph.D.

Personal

Born May 18, 1921, Reading, Pennsylvania
Married: Vallie Moyer, Reading; 1 child

Education

1953 Pennsylvania State University, B.S., Microbiology, Honors
1954 University of Wisconsin, M.S., Microbiology, WARF Fellow
1958 Pennsylvania State University, Ph.D., Microbiology

Experience Teaching and Research

1953–1954 Research Assistant, University of Wisconsin
1954–1958 Instructor, Pennsylvania State University
1958–1960 Instructor, University of Illinois, College of Medicine
1960–1961 Instructor, Johns Hopkins University, School of Hygiene
1961–1962 Assistant Professor, Johns Hopkins University
1960–1962 Associate Microbiologist, Leonard Wood Memorial
1962–1983 Microbiologist, Leonard Wood Memorial

1963–1983 Laboratory Director, Leonard Wood Memorial
1964–1970 Chief, Laboratory Branch, Leonard Wood Memorial
1965–1980 Assistant Professor, Johns Hopkins University, School of Hygiene
1972–1983 Chief of Operations, Leonard Wood Memorial
1980——Professor Microbiology, George Washington University
1983——Emeritus Chief of Operations, Leonard Wood Memorial

Professional Societies

American Association for the Advancement of Science
American Society of Microbiology
American Academy of Microbiology
Conference of Research Workers in Animal Diseases
Cebu Medical Society, Philippine Medical Association
International Leprosy Association
New York Academy of Science
Sigma Xi

Supplementary Information

Special Consultant, World Health Organization, Geneva
Member, Leprosy Expert Panel, World Health Organization
Scientific Advisory Committee, College San Jose de Recoletos
John A. Hartford Foundation, Research Award, Bacteriology of Leprosy, 1970
Scientific Advisory Board, International Leprosy Center, Caracas

Consultant, Pan American Health Organization
World Health Organization Research Grant in Leprosy 1970–1979
John A. Hartford Foundation Research Award for Leprosy 1974–1977
Principal Investigator, National Institute of Health, Contract No. AI-52509
Principal Investigator, Research Grant Sovereign Military Order of Malta
Administrator Research Grant Sasakawa Memorial Health Foundation, Tokyo
Reading Senior High School Alumni Association Hall of Fame
Companion of Merit and Bronze Medal of Honor, Military and Hospitaller Order St. Lazarus of Jerusalem
The Torch Club, Reading

Epilogue

Mrs. Tony Madarang, Monina, was my administrative assistant. She served as my right hand for most of my professional life in Cebu. It was only her continuation as chief executive officer when I left Cebu, and the knowledge that the laboratory that I had created was in good hands, that allowed me to accept retirement without putting up a significant struggle.

We remained in constant contact by letter, cable and phone for many years after my retirement. In one of my letters, in response to her request, I sent her a passage from this book of memories of Cebu that I had told her I was writing. The passage that I sent was the last paragraph of this book, about the fading memory blossoms. She never mentioned it in any of her later letters, nor did I ask.

Some time in mid 1987, I got a letter from Mother Rictrude, one of the nuns in the leprosarium. She wrote that Monina was rapidly dying from terminal cancer. Mother's letter confirmed what I had heard at least a year earlier. Neither Monina nor I ever mentioned this in any of our correspondence. She continued to administer the laboratory from her bed at home until her death.

In December of 1987, Tony and Monina called me while she was on her deathbed in Cebu. We spoke, long distance, for almost an hour during which she told me, in tears, that she couldn't write to me about my blossoms from the kalatuchi tree. It made her too sad. She died several days later. The last thing she had said to me was, "I will see you again."

Almost two years later in December 1989, I received a note and a check for a rather large amount of money from Tony. In the note, Tony wrote that he was sending the money as a dying request from Monina, that I was to buy myself a piece of the crystal glassware that she knew I loved.

The Steuben crystal piece is beyond my description. I see it every day. The sad memories of the fading blossoms from the kalatuchi tree have been replaced by the lasting beauty of the crystal "Peony Bowl."

Last week, February 15, 1990, Mother Rictrude wrote about the kalatuchi tree, " . . . they are in full bloom now with the heat that is coming up. . . . "

I honestly thought that this was the time of the year that the kalatuchi rested.